WHAT TO DO WHEN THE DOCTOR SAYS IT'S

PCOS

WHAT TO DO WHEN THE DOCTOR SAYS IT'S

PCOS

MILTON HAMMERLY, M.D.
and CHERYL KIMBALL

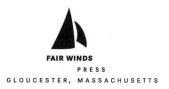

FAIR WINDS
PRESS
GLOUCESTER, MASSACHUSETTS

Text ©2003 Milton Hammerly, M.D., and Cheryl Kimball

First published in the USA in 2003 by
Fair Winds Press
33 Commercial Street
Gloucester, MA 01930

Library of Congress Cataloging-in-Publication Data available

ISBN 1-59233-004-5

10 9 8 7 6 5 4 3 2 1

Cover design: Laura Shaw Design
Book design: *tabula rasa* graphic design

Printed and bound in Canada

The information in this book is for educational purposes only.
It is not intended to replace the advice of a physician or medical
practitioner. Please see your health care provider before beginning
any new health program.

CONTENTS

FOREWORD

Polycystic ovarian syndrome—It's a mouthful to say. The name itself can be confusing to the listener, since it inadequately and misleadingly describes the condition as a seemingly physiological "female problem." Even medical professionals often do not understand what it is. When spoken in general conversation, this term elicits a blank stare from most people. Others nod knowingly, as they mistakenly assume this condition is related to development of classic "ovarian cysts," a common but usually unrelated gynecological condition.

What most do not know is that PCOS is an important endocrine condition, affecting many hormones throughout a woman's body, and impacting multiple organ systems and metabolic processes. It manifests itself in a diverse set of symptoms that are seemingly unrelated. Yet all of these symptoms are very much a part of the same condition, a condition that must be treated. But how?

In 1996, I learned from an online infertility discussion forum that a syndrome known as PCOS might explain the set of symptoms that I had experienced throughout my own life. I set out to learn everything I could about this syndrome. I downed many cups of gourmet coffee while diligently searching the computer systems at the local Barnes & Noble and Borders bookstores. I made extensive use of the then-fledgling Amazon.com online search functionality. And what was the fruit of my effort? I found almost nothing. I located one 2-inch thick book on women's health, which contained one scrawny paragraph on PCOS. The extent of that paragraph was to describe the appearance of the polycystic ovary, and its possible association to irregular menstrual periods. I needed a book to help me understand this syndrome! Yet there was no book to be found.

Since there was so little information on PCOS, I assumed that it must be a very rare condition. I suspected I was one of a handful of women in the world who were afflicted with this mysterious and frustrating syndrome. Only when I began to search through medical journals and read research studies did I learn that the prevalence of PCOS was at least 5 percent of the female population. I was stunned!

How could a condition that is so common, be accompanied by a total void in patient information and educational materials? In this era of "self-help" resources, where were the books that could help me to learn what this condition was, and what I could do about it? How was I supposed to learn what was "normal," and what might be different about me? There were plenty of books on endometriosis, fibroids, various kinds of cancer, depression; the list went on. But what about PCOS? Where could I turn for help?

I only wish that, back in 1996, I had the book you are about to read. I needed to learn about my own body. What was happening? Why had I gained so much weight? Why didn't I have ovulatory menstrual cycles? Why did I have hair growing on my face and other places that I didn't want anyone to know about? And why did I have cystic acne all along my jaw line? And most importantly, what were my options for treatment? My doctors didn't know anything about this syndrome. They had never diagnosed or even mentioned it.

I was amazed to learn, through reading medical journals, that PCOS was nothing new and could be easily identified in many patients with "classic" symptoms. I approached one of the clinical researchers whose PCOS study I had read, and requested evaluation for PCOS. The diagnosis was a slam-dunk. So why, over the course of my adult life, did 13 doctors of various disciplines completely miss the diagnosis? It became clear to me that I would need to take the driver's seat in attending to my own health care. But I also wanted to help others avoid the frustration I had encountered in my attempts to learn about PCOS. I wanted to help others sit in that driver's seat as well.

I began an online PCOS discussion in an infertility forum. I immediately learned that there were many women just like me, within the infertility support group, who suffered from PCOS and also felt that they were alone. Most had very little knowledge on the condition, and felt that their doctors didn't understand it either. With the technical help of some of the forum members, we were able to begin a discussion forum dedicated to PCOS, and expanding beyond the infertility aspects of the condition. How did PCOS affect teenagers? What happened to women with PCOS after menopause? What was the connection between insulin and PCOS? What should we be eating? What medications might work? There were still many unanswered questions.

The group was a success. Women helped other women to get answers to questions. Some of the information shared was good information. Other information was not necessarily accurate. But regardless, information was flowing. Soon it became clear that a central, formal organization was needed. The quality of information that was disseminated needed to undergo scrutiny and an approval process for accuracy and appropriateness. There was a voice that needed to be heard, and a constituency to be served. So we planned a conference, and invited the best researchers and speakers on PCOS that we could find. The Polycystic Ovarian Syndrome Association (PCOSA, www.pcosupport.org) was born from that conference in May 1997.

The journey has come full-circle now. Over the past five years, through programming, online resources and print publications, PCOSA has often been the starting point for the education of both patients and doctors on the subject on PCOS. And sometimes, even writers find that the information and resources that PCOSA offers can be of assistance in writing the very kind of book that I needed so desperately in 1996. I could not thank Dr. Milton Hammerly and Cheryl Kimball more for writing this book.

It is this type of guide that sheds light on the many mysteries the PCOS patient strives to solve in her journey toward achieving her best possible health and quality of life. Management of PCOS requires active decisions on the part of the patient, and an understanding of all points of view and options will best prepare her for those decisions. I hope that this book will inform you, prepare you, and inspire you to sit in the driver's seat as you seek the best possible care for "your" PCOS, and that it helps you to achieve your best possible health and quality of life.

Christine Gray DeZarn, Founder
Polycystic Ovarian Syndrome Association, Inc. (PCOSA)

INTRODUCTION

Curse or Blessing?

Do you have irregular menstrual cycles, unwanted facial hair growth, male-pattern hair loss, acne, unexplained weight gain, and infertility? Have you resigned yourself, out of sheer frustration, to putting up with these symptoms after being told repeatedly by multiple physicians that there's nothing wrong? If so, chances are pretty good that you may have polycystic ovarian syndrome (PCOS). Even if you don't want children and don't mind plucking, there are a number of things you can and should do to treat this condition.

PCOS can actually be an early warning sign for more serious problems that should not be ignored. The underlying cause of PCOS in many women seems to be insulin resistance, and up to 40 percent will go on to develop impaired glucose tolerance or full-blown diabetes by the age of forty. Strange as it may seem, the curse of PCOS can also be a blessing, since men have no comparable early warning system to alert them that they are on the road to diabetes and all its associated potential complications.

Common but Rare

Does a tree falling in the forest make any noise if nobody is there to hear it? Does a common medical disorder get the attention it deserves if physicians don't diagnose it?

Such is the paradox of polycystic ovarian syndrome. PCOS is the most common hormonal disorder among women of reproductive age, affecting about 6 percent of this group. Based on statistics from the U.S. 2000 Census, there are approximately 80 million women of reproductive age, which means that, of these, roughly 4.8 million have PCOS.

Why is it, then, that the National Organization for Rare Disorders (NORD), which focuses on disorders affecting fewer than 200,000 people in the United States, has labeled PCOS a rare disorder? Is it possible that PCOS is so underdiagnosed (200,000 out of 4.8 million suggests that only one out of twenty-four women with this condition is actually being diagnosed) that this common condition could be mischaracterized as rare?

Twin Epidemics

Diabetes, which you never hear characterized as rare, affects about 6 percent of the U.S. population. The increasing incidence of diabetes in the U.S. (thought to be in large part related to our affluent lifestyle, associated with too many calories consumed and not enough physical activity) has been called an epidemic with tremendous public health implications. Diabetes dramatically increases the risk of a number of serious conditions, including heart disease, kidney failure, blindness, nerve damage, and amputations, to name a few.

PCOS, which uncoincidentally has an incidence comparable to diabetes in women of reproductive age, is a twin to diabetes. As the incidence of diabetes increases, so will the incidence of PCOS, and vice versa. PCOS can be thought of as a potentially "prediabetic" stage that offers an opportunity to both know and change the future. While knowing and changing the future sounds like the stuff of science fiction, it is also one of the most basic tenets of preventive medicine. This simple understanding, if applied, could dramatically improve efforts to prevent and control diabetes in women.

So why is PCOS so common and yet so rarely diagnosed? Is PCOS somehow difficult to diagnose? The answers to these questions can be found in both the history of the disorder and trends in medical education.

A Medical Mystery?

When first discovered by Drs. Stein and Leventhal over seventy years ago, the condition was, not surprisingly, named Stein-Leventhal syndrome. One of the earlier treatments was "wedge resection" of the ovaries to remove the abnormal cysts that are present in many (but not all) women with this condition. Unfortunately, since the cysts are not the cause of the problem, wedge resection may not be helpful. Following on the heels of the "anatomic" phase of PCOS (thinking in terms of an anatomic cause and cure) came the "reproductive endocrine" phase. The reproductive endocrine phase is typified by thinking that PCOS is caused entirely by an imbalance in the hormonal signaling between the hypothalamus, the pituitary gland, and the ovaries. This imbalance was thought to cause the decrease in estrogen levels and increase in male hormones seen in patients with PCOS. Treatments based on the reproductive endocrine understanding have sought to alter the imbalanced pituitary and ovarian hormones through the use of medications. Since the reproductive endocrine understanding is closer to the truth than the anatomic one, these hormonal manipulations have proven more beneficial than wedge resection.

The most current understanding of PCOS can be described as the "endocrine network" phase. Decreased sensitivity to insulin, the major hormone responsible for regulating blood sugar, often seems to amplify or be responsible for the alterations in hypothalamic, pituitary gland, and ovarian signaling. The latest research indicates that PCOS is not simply abnormal ovaries or abnormal signaling between the pituitary and ovarian glands, but rather a complex network of hormonal interactions and disruptions in which insulin resistance plays a major role.

While the scientific understanding of PCOS has clearly evolved through different stages, its name is still an outdated tribute to the

anatomic understanding of this condition. The mere label of PCOS
is thus a barrier to better understanding of this disease. Another barrier has been the historical trend in medical education to organize
training according to isolated organs and systems rather than complex
interactive networks. Perhaps it's time to rename this disorder in order
to enhance a better understanding among both medical practitioners
and the general population. "Insulin Resistant Ovarian Syndrome"
(IROS) might work, but it implies that insulin resistance and the
ovaries are the only problems. "Insulin Resistant Female Endocrine
Network Dysfunction" (IRFEND), though cumbersome, gives a more
balanced perspective. Medical mysteries, somewhat like mystery nov-
els, are solved when you search for clues, scrutinize suspects, and determine whodunit. IRFEND takes away the mystery by succinctly
summarizing the scientific clues and pointing us in the direction of the
most likely suspects. Grasping this makes the diagnosis quite simple;
the challenge is in calling it by the right name so that people will think
of it in the right way.

An Unconventional Non-Departure From Convention
While I was at first tempted to genuflect at the altar of convention
to avoid confusion, if conventional labels are in fact the cause of
confusion, I would only be perpetuating confusion by continuing to
use outdated and obsolete terminology. Therefore my second temptation was to dispense with PCOS and only refer to IRFEND for the
remainder of this book. If we want to give PCOS/IRFEND the
recognition and attention it deserves in the medical community and
the general population, a good place to start is by giving it the right
name! However, realizing that IRFEND doesn't exactly flow off the
lips and that greater minds than mine will probably come up with a
more suitable and catchy name, it would be presumptuous and needlessly disruptive to insist on the supremacy of a temporary label that
will come and go.

As a result of these mental gymnastics, I have chosen, for the purposes of this book, to stick with the conventional term of PCOS, even though it is abundantly clear that the terminology needs to be changed. Until the name of PCOS is officially changed, let us remain fully and constantly aware of its shortcomings and the hurdles it puts up in the way of better understanding.

Hope Amidst the Confusion

Even though the PCOS label creates confusion, we now know much more than we ever did about this disorder. Every woman with PCOS is different and, as a result, treatments need to be individualized to get the best possible results. In this book you will find explanations of the most current knowledge, many effective treatments, and suggestions on how to best tailor interventions to your unique situation.

We know that PCOS affects far more than just the ovaries. PCOS touches the body, mind, and spirit of patients afflicted by this condition. To ignore this reality by simply suggesting that the latest medications will cure this disease would be unrealistic and a disservice. By embracing the interconnectedness of body, mind, and spirit, this book offers you hope for today and for the future. PCOS offers a rare opportunity to see the future and change it through lifestyle changes augmented with complementary therapies and medicines, if needed. Looking through the window of PCOS, we see an abundance of hope, knowing that the symptoms of today can be managed and the complications of tomorrow can be prevented.

CHAPTER ONE ∿

Defining PCOS
What Is It, and What Does It Do to My Body?

Mention polycystic ovarian syndrome to most people, and you will most likely be greeted by a blank stare. However, despite the lack of common knowledge about PCOS, the syndrome, according to the Mayo Clinic, is "the most common hormonal disorder among women of reproductive age in the United States, affecting an estimated 4 percent to 12 percent."

To give a definitive diagnosis, the National Institutes of Health (NIH) came up with a set of three criteria that a woman must exhibit to be considered a PCOS patient. They are:

1. *Irregular or absence of menstruation:* Young women and their doctors often dismiss irregular periods as a common occurrence, as a girl's body adjusts to the onset of menses. Thus, the irregularity of a woman's menstrual cycles is often not considered

a medical issue until she is at a stage in her life when she is attempting to start a family. The regularity or irregularity of cycles can be determined through anecdotal evidence by you, the patient.

2. *Excess androgens (male hormones that are normally present in small amounts in females):* Male hormones are naturally present in women's bodies; however, women with PCOS may experience excess male hormones that result in difficult symptoms such as male-pattern hair growth, acne, and male-pattern baldness. A blood test can determine the level of male hormones.

3. *Lack of other reasons for the above two symptoms:* Many reasons exist for a woman to have irregular menstrual periods, and many things can be the cause of an imbalance of hormones, from tumors to hypothyroidism (which slows down the protein that binds estrogen and testosterone) to hyperprolactinemia (an excess of the hormone that produces breast milk and suppresses ovulation).

These three criteria are simply the conditions by which PCOS is diagnosed. There are many other symptoms experienced by women with PCOS, many of which can be much more frustrating and health-impairing than these three.

Ironically, the symptom that is not on this list, and that is generally not only the least annoying but also unconnected to most health problems, is the very symptom that gives the disease its name: multiple cysts on the ovaries. The polycystic ovary is detected via ultrasound, often as a confirmation but not a diagnostic test. Many women who have been diagnosed with PCOS, and are being treated for it, never have it confirmed whether their ovaries have cysts or not.

PCO vs. PCOS

The preceeding criteria mean that a woman can have polycystic ovaries but not have polycystic ovarian syndrome. Without the presence of those three criteria, the ovary with multiple cysts does not automatically mean a PCOS diagnosis. Although it may be implicated in difficulty getting pregnant, the cystic ovary itself rarely causes any overt problems that would send a woman to the doctor.

It is those overt problems that initiate a doctor visit, and suggest a diagnosis of PCOS. Once PCOS is suspected, the ovaries may be ultrasounded to confirm whether they have cysts on them or not, but it is not even necessary at that stage, since, as you will recall, the three NIH criteria do not include cysts on the ovaries.

On the other hand, women who meet the three criteria leading to a PCOS diagnosis almost invariably have polycystic ovaries, although there are even exceptions to that.

Armed with a Diagnosis

If you have been diagnosed with polycystic ovarian syndrome, be comforted by the fact that at least now, with a diagnosis, you can start making some progress in alleviating your symptoms. Many PCOS sufferers experience symptoms for years before figuring out what is going on. The symptoms of PCOS seem so wildly disparate from one woman to another, and each woman's individual symptoms seemed so unrelated to each other that, until the past few years, the disorder was often not considered in an attempt to diagnose a woman's problems. Instead, the problems were often attributed to the symptoms themselves—infertility was simply the reason one couldn't get pregnant; the inability to stay on a diet and eat right caused the weight issues; oily skin or poor nutrition was blamed for acne, long after the teen acne years had passed.

PCOS diagnosis can indeed be elusive. Symptoms often seem disconnected, and one symptom itself rarely sends the woman to a doctor in search of a cause—except perhaps in the case of infertility. Some of the symptoms are so overwhelming that others may be overlooked. A woman may be so focused on trying to take care of, say, obesity that she may not notice, or may not give too much thought to, symptoms that are less of a cosmetic or health issue, such as an irregular menstrual cycle. Her cycle's irregularities may not mean anything to her until she begins to try to get pregnant. So, PCOS can escape her or her doctor's radar screen for quite some time before it is considered as a possible problem.

On the other hand, some women may show polycystic ovaries—the very source of the name of the syndrome—but never exhibit the symptoms of the syndrome itself. So, ovaries with many cysts do not immediately indicate PCOS.

It's Not Just the Way Things Are

If a woman lives an average lifespan of eighty years, she spends about half of her life—from age twelve to fifty-plus—experiencing the monthly cycle of menstruation. Then several years are usually devoted to menopause and coping with the varying degrees of severity with which her body experiences significant hormonal changes, and the other changes they cause in her appearance and emotions. No wonder women are accustomed to simply dealing with things like the symptoms presented by PCOS! You miss a few periods, you gain a few pounds that you can't seem to shed, you're fatigued a lot of the time—that's a woman's life, right? Not!

Often, a woman assumes that this is simply how her body operates. She may be suffering from polycystic ovarian syndrome without knowing it, while she is concentrating on trying to lose weight, embarrassed by having to shave excess body hair, and depressed by the feeling that her body doesn't cooperate, no matter how hard she tries.

But if a woman's body is functioning as nature intended, she does not have to consider these things "normal." PCOS and its symptoms are not normal, and as we come to understand more about this previously mysterious collection of symptoms, we find more evidence pointing to things women can do to turn their symptoms around.

Periods

Light, short, irregular periods are not the way a woman's reproductive system is set up to function, as you will read in further detail in Chapter Two, "The Way It Is Meant to Be." There is a natural cycle that a woman's body goes through during the reproductive years of her life. In order for her to get pregnant, these processes must happen. They include movement of an egg into position to be successfully fertilized by a sperm (ovulation), developing a lining in the uterus to accommodate the development of that egg into a fetus and baby, and shedding of that lining if a certain amount of time passes and it becomes clear that this cycle's egg is not going to be fertilized (menstruation).

Understandably, women who experience short menstrual cycles with light blood flow, or even skip monthly periods, are often not too quick to complain! However, when a woman with abnormal menstruation tries to become pregnant, she will seek medical help. This explains why many women with PCOS are diagnosed through the fertility clinic channel.

If this same woman is overweight, she may have accepted the fact that she is just "designed that way" or that she doesn't really have the discipline to "eat right." She may experience adult acne but, since she's overweight and has decided she doesn't/can't eat right, she assumes that the acne must be connected to that. The cycle continues until it is disrupted by something specific like a blood test showing thyroid problems, or, again, her inability to get pregnant.

A Couple of Important Clarifications
Polycystic ovarian syndrome is often considered by women, and treated by their doctors, as a reproductive disorder. The classic reason for this is that PCOS is typically first discovered in women when they wind up at a fertility clinic because they are having difficulty getting pregnant. The disorder is often characterized by—and was named for—numerous cysts lining the outer edge of the ovaries. This so-called "string of pearls" is thought to be caused by egg follicles (the cellular complexes that surround and nurture the egg in the ovary) collecting in the ovary as a result of the lack of ovulation that most PCOS sufferers experience. Normally, the egg would pass through the system unfertilized.

But the reproductive issues women with PCOS experience are caused by hormonal imbalances, making polycystic ovarian syndrome not a reproductive disorder but an endocrine (relating to hormones) disorder. Once you are diagnosed with PCOS, the next specialist you should turn to is an endocrinologist.

Although we have just been hearing more about it in the past five years or so, polycystic ovarian syndrome (PCOS) is far from a newcomer to the women's health scene. The syndrome is also called Stein-Leventhal sydrome, named for two doctors—Irving Stein and Michael Leventhal—who began to diagnose PCOS back in 1935. In fact, in the late 1990s, Dr. Sarah H. Wild released the results of a study she did of 786 women with PCOS. The group of women in her study had a mean age of twenty-five years, and Dr. Wild followed them for thirty-two years. While the knowledge of PCOS is not old in relative terms, it is also not something that just cropped up in women in the past couple of years.

But syndromes, by definition, are more complicated and harder to diagnose than specific diseases, which typically have a specific cause and effect. PCOS is not a terminal illness in itself, nor is it communicable, so it has not enjoyed the extensive and intensive research that other diseases have been given—even though it is considered the most common endocrine disorder that women face. In fact, recent statistics cited by Timothy Kirn in *Family Practice News* (August 15, 2002) show that 6 percent of women in the U.S. have PCOS.

A woman who complains of the sometimes seemingly unrelated symptoms that a syndrome can present is often made to feel that she is a hypochondriac and that she should perhaps suffer in silence and take care of these "minor" issues in the best way she can. After all, women are supposed to deal with all these issues, right? Absolutely wrong!

This Book's for You

While perhaps an occasional cramp or irregular period is unavoidable and therefore considered "normal" in women, there is no reason for women to suffer the list of symptoms that can be displayed by the person with PCOS. Weight gain, adult acne, head hair loss, and excessive facial hair are not things that a woman should have to experience if her body is functioning as it was designed to do. Simple as that. And those are just the annoying symptoms.

PCOS can also bring symptoms that can lead to life-threatening problems. Because of the underlying hormonal causes of PCOS symptoms, women are typically suffering PCOS during the years when they would like to be having children, so that the inability to become pregnant is yet another major issue.

Top all this off with the depression that results from dealing with all of these symptoms, and you have a problem that women need to control. This book will help you sort through all the pieces and determine where you need to focus your efforts.

Although things are changing quickly, there is not yet much out there on PCOS that is immediately accessible to the millions of women worldwide who suffer with the disorder. With this book, we hope to help you make some sense of your disorder and the specifics of your experience with it. We will guide you through what is going on in your body, in terms you can understand. We will give you the latest information and the resources to check for updating your knowledge. You will learn how your body is intended to function, what effect PCOS is having, and the things you can do.

Although working with your OB/GYN, fertility specialist, dermatologist, and endocrinologist is critical to your success in dealing with PCOS, this disorder is by nature one in which the patient needs to take control of her own well-being. Be sure to keep a personal record of your progress with specific symptoms. In this book you will find tips on weight loss, skin care, and hair care. We also bring in the mental health issue with some tips on how to pump up your self-esteem and combat the depression that can accompany a chronic disorder especially one like PCOS, where even the medical community is still sorting out important details and treatment options.

In this book you will also find a dozen case studies of women who have PCOS. Although their syndrome may be the same, PCOS sufferers each experience a very different disorder. Their stories may help you understand some of your own symptoms better. We hope you will also take comfort in knowing that other people have successfully dealt with many of the same things you are experiencing.

What Is a Syndrome?

Unlike a disease, which has a specific pathological origin, a syndrome is a condition that exists only as a collection of symptoms. Consider cystic fibrosis, a disease that causes the body to produce an unnaturally large amount of sticky mucous, resulting in long-term deterioration of the lungs, as well as other conditions related to mucous production. The disease is present when a person receives a specific gene from both parents. The genes are the cause, the excess mucous production is the effect, and the lung deterioration and a few other conditons are the symptoms. The symptoms are specific to the disease and lead to the specific diagnosis.

A syndrome is not a specific disease like cystic fibrosis, diabetes, or Alzheimer's. It is a collection of symptoms; typically, at least a certain number of symptoms must be present for someone to be diagnosed with the syndrome. Perhaps each symptom could lead to a specific disease, but it doesn't. The symptoms of PCOS are not diseases in and of themselves, but in conjunction they lead to a diagnosis of the syndrome.

What Are the Symptoms of PCOS?

Women with polycystic ovarian syndrome have several—often seemingly unrelated—symptoms, many of which appear to be merely cosmetic annoyances. In Chapters Three and Four, we will go into each of the PCOS symptoms in more detail, but here is a list of the possible symptoms of the syndrome. Please keep in mind that PCOS patients rarely experience *all* of these symptoms! Also, if you have one or two of these symptoms, it does not automatically mean that you have PCOS.

A patient with PCOS may experience:
• Obesity
• Amenorrhea (absence of menstruation)
• Oligomenorrhea (light and infrequent menstrual flow)

- Hirsutism (abnormal/excessive hair growth)
- Oily skin
- Acne
- Abnormal vaginal bleeding
- Infertility
- Recurrent miscarriage
- Alopecia (hair loss/baldness)
- Acrochordons (skin tags)
- Anovulation (absence of ovulation)
- Depression

Other symptoms that show up in the process of diagnosis, from a blood test and other testing, include:
- Cysts on the ovaries
- Elevated testosterone level
- Elevated insulin level
- Insulin resistance (failure of the cells to respond to insulin)
- Elevated luteinizing hormone
- Depressed sex-hormone-binding globulin (SHBG)
- Abnormal lipid profile

All of these symptoms will be discussed in more detail in later chapters as well as in the personal stories at the end of each chapter.

Just What Exactly Is Happening?

The textbook case of PCOS shows ovaries with a ring of cysts around the edge. These cysts are under the surface and show up as small bumps. They are not the same as "ovarian cysts," which (1) are typically found within the ovary, (2) occur singly, not as a group, (3) can grow larger—and can reduce—in size, and (4) have the ability to interfere with the normal function of the ovary.

The classic PCOS ring of cysts is not the cause of the syndrome, and in fact is not always present in PCOS patients; the ring of cysts is simply another symptom. This contributes to the reasoning that surgical removal of these cysts would do nothing to relieve the syndrome.

The cysts are thought to be caused by follicles collected when the ovary doesn't go on to release an egg. The cysts are typically numerous, ten or more, and very small. Because of their number and placement around the outer edge of the ovary, surgical removal is not considered useful and would in fact require significant removal of the ovary tissue, which could damage the ovary and cause it to no longer function. Chapter Five, "Medical Treatment for PCOS: Drugs and Surgical Options," discusses this in more detail.

If the cysts are just another symptom, what is really at the root of PCOS? It is, ultimately, suspected to be an inherited genetic disorder. According to Dr. Yaron Tomer of the Mt. Sinai School of Medicine (quoted by Bruce Jancin in the August 15, 2000, issue of *Family Practice News*), "A susceptibility gene for PCOS appears to be on chromosome 19 near the insulin receptor gene."

The Root Cause

If the cysts and weight gain and hair loss and acne and fatigue and depression are just symptoms, then what is causing them? What is really going on in the body of a woman with PCOS?

This is the part that is beginning to become more clear. The actual process that triggers the syndrome and its symptoms is linked to a hormonal imbalance in the endocrine system, specifically involving the hormone insulin. This imbalance is the underlying cause of the symptoms exhibited by a PCOS patient, all of which can be traced to the function of hormones in the body. Insulin resistance (failure of the cells to respond to normal amounts of insulin) and hyperinsulinemia (too much insulin in the bloodstream) are thought to be the main issues.

As explained by Jennifer Couzin in the November 5, 2001, issue of *Newsweek*, "Many PCOS women do not respond properly to insulin; when they eat a meal, the insulin released by the pancreas isn't enough to move glucose into cells the way it's supposed to, so the body keeps pumping out more hormone." This insulin connection makes PCOS a major risk factor in contracting type 2 diabetes.

One of these hormonal imbalances occurs because the ovaries are not producing hormones in the proportions that the body is designed for. This in turn causes other hormone—releasing organs, such as the pituitary gland, to gauge incorrectly the amount of hormones to release—and a vicious cycle results. If all organs are doing their job properly, everything works smoothly. But as with any syndrome, disease, injury, or other contributor to malfunction in the body, when one thing goes wrong, many others are affected.

This chain-of-events scenario can be very hard to deal with, but the key is to attack the problem at the beginning of the chain. This in turn impacts the links all along the way, hopefully pulling the whole chain back on track.

Things You Will Hear Often in Conjunction with PCOS
When you research and talk with medical professionals about PCOS, there are several things you will hear about often. They include:

> *Insulin resistance:* When the cells in your body are resistant to insulin, the body produces more insulin in order to try to get its message across. The pancreas, which produces insulin, is not designed to keep up with this abnormal demand.

Hyperinsulinemia: The prefix "hyper" simply means "excessive." So, hyperinsulinemia means excessive amounts of insulin in the bloodstream, a direct result of insulin resistance. The insulin connection with PCOS is fascinating and has been the source of much speculation and study as to the root cause of PCOS. Excessive insulin elevates testosterone and causes the liver to reduce its production of SHBG (sex-hormone-binding globulin), which causes a dysfunction in how the body responds to the male and female sex hormones. This complex chain of events starts to explain some of the androgenous (masculine) characteristics of PCOS symptoms. Despite these evident connections, however, no exact cause of PCOS has been discovered with certainty.

Impaired fasting glucose: When you eat, insulin rushes to the scene to transform the glucose to energy or store it in the form of fat. Impaired fasting glucose refers to a high level of glucose in a fasting person, which indicates insulin resistance.

Impaired glucose tolerance: This is typical of insulin resistance. When the pancreas can no longer produce enough insulin to meet the excessive demands of the insulin-resistant cells, glucose levels in the body spike, especially after eating when the demand on the pancreas is greatest.

Follicle-stimulating hormone (FSH): This hormone stimulates the follicles in the ovaries to produce eggs. The pituitary gland is responsible for releasing FSH.

Endocrinology: The endocrine system secretes the hormones that tell the body what to do. Endocrinology is the study of the endocrine system. PCOS patients are well advised to have an endocrinologist on their medical team.

The role of carbohydrates: Carbohydrates are the food source that insulin reacts to. Diets designed for people with diabetes balance carbohydrate intake.

Central obesity: Central obesity refers to the type of profile of an overweight woman that is described as "apple-shaped" (as opposed to "pear-shaped"). Insulin resistance is often the cause of this weight distribution.

What to Do?

As you will see in the chapters following, treating PCOS is a multifaceted process. Focusing on exercise and diet combined with your doctor's prescribed regimen of drug therapy, and perhaps some alternative therapies, is the path to dealing with PCOS. Yes, it is a lot of work, but we are all dealt some cards that we have no control over, and your health is worth the extra work!

Some women choose to ignore PCOS. As you will read in the stories that accompany each of the chapters in this book, some women are just too busy with families to spend the considerable time it takes to focus on their own health. While this is understandable and simply a reality for some women at some point in their lives, it is probably not best for you or your family.

PCOS symptoms can make a woman pretty miserable. If you are feeling down and discouraged about your own health, you may think you are ignoring it, but you probably aren't. You may not realize how much joy you are taking out of your own day just by not tackling these issues. You may get irritable with your family—mood swings and irritability are associated with PCOS, a common side effect of hormonal imbalances.

While most PCOS symptoms are not life-threatening, there are some elements of the disorder that are significant health issues. The link of PCOS to diabetes is one of the most important ones—women with PCOS are more prone to developing short-term gestational and long-term type 2 (also known as "adult onset" or noninsulin-dependent) diabetes.

According to Mayo Clinic reports, women with PCOS also experience more imbalances of "good" vs. "bad" cholesterol, giving them an increased risk of coronary artery disease, as well as high blood pressure.

These potential threats alone should help you decide it is time to attack the problem. Also, if you are so committed to raising your children that you can't take time away from them to concentrate on your own health, what kind of message are you sending them about the importance of taking care of themselves, and the benefits of good health care?

Other Serious Risk Factors

As if that isn't enough, there are several other serious risk factors associated with PCOS and its symptoms. We mentioned above diabetes, coronary artery disease, and high blood pressure. PCOS patients are also at risk for endometrial cancer, a precancerous condition known as endometrial hyperplasia, and other endometrial disease associated with long-term irregular cycles and the lack of the natural shedding of the uterine lining. According to the International Council on Infertility Information Dissemination, the risk is greater for those who have fewer than one menstrual period every three months—in other words, when the uterine lining regularly goes longer than three months without being shed.

Interrelated Symptoms

One of the more complicating factors of PCOS is that it consists of a group of interrelated symptoms, which can make dealing with it as frustrating as trying to determine which came first, the chicken or the egg. Obesity, for instance, is known to exacerbate many of the other symptoms of PCOS—insulin resistance is greater in overweight individuals, other hormone levels are greatly affected by weight, menstruation can be thrown off by being over or under what is considered optimal weight for your height and body type.

As you are attempting to regulate cycles and address infertility, medications can add to your weight control problems. Women with extreme symptoms of PCOS can become depressed, and depression means that they are less likely to follow through with the complex process of trying to control symptoms and especially to lose weight.

PCOS can be a difficult cycle of cause and effect. You need to get into the best frame of mind possible to take control of your body and get the syndrome in check. As you will find out throughout this book, it's a lot of work, but it is definitely possible!

Working with Your Doctor

Later chapters will deal with the specifics of working with your health professionals—and if you decide to deal with PCOS, you will definitely be working with more than one health professional. But suffice it to say here that, perhaps even more than with other aspects of your health care, you need to be proactive about your treatment. You do need to:

- Be honest and upfront with your doctor about the type and severity of your symptoms.

- Educate yourself through all means possible, not only about the intricacies of PCOS itself, but also about all the various symptoms and possible treatments.

- Learn to be confident in speaking with your doctor.

Do what your health care professionals recommend, if you want the treatment of PCOS to actually accomplish something. You can't go just halfway with treatment recommendations, then complain that the regimen isn't helping, and stop treatment. Stick with it!

The current generation of women in the age group to be experiencing PCOS may not need this advice, but beware of the "doctor as God" trap. Don't assume that she or he knows best, and think, "Who am I to say?" This is your body, your life, and the things that you need to deal with. Doctors are not mind readers, and they do take your information and input seriously. They want you to care about your treatment and to feel that you are in the driver's seat when it comes to your health. If you don't, then the doctor can talk and dispense advice and prescriptions and a plan, but all of it will do no good if it seems that you aren't going to follow it anyway.

One final note about working with your doctor: The symptoms of PCOS are also symptoms that relate to many other diseases and conditions. Don't assume you have PCOS and treat yourself; work with your doctor to get a firm diagnosis. The insulin connection of PCOS makes it very similar to diabetes, and literally dozens of things could cause fertility issues. Some symptoms can be caused by life-threatening medical issues or can turn into life-threatening medical issues if they aren't properly diagnosed.

PCOS in Teens

PCOS as a syndrome doesn't just suddenly appear. It is a dysfunction of the endocrine system, and if it is truly a genetic disorder, it is there within the body all of a woman's life. In young women, PCOS may not exhibit in clear-cut ways. Teens are moving through many hormonal changes in the body's journey to childbearing capabilities, and many of the classic PCOS symptoms—irregular periods, weight issues, acne—are often accepted as part of the process of growing up. So PCOS can hang out incognito in the young woman's body for quite a few years.

Often not until the teen reaches adult age and is still experiencing irregular menstruation, acne, and other "adolescent problems" does she become suspicious of what's going on. Top that off with the inability to start a family, and that is when the PCOS sufferer finally finds herself at the doctor and, ultimately, the fertility clinic. And if she's very lucky, the term PCOS comes up.

Don't Get Discouraged Now!

Many women interviewed for this book mentioned that when they told friends and family members about their PCOS diagnosis, they were looked at askance—PCOS is not a disorder that many people have heard of. Yet.

Another syndrome, known as fibromyalgia, causes chronic pain that interferes with restful sleep, resulting in another of those vicious cycles. Until just a few years ago, it was an obscure collection of symptoms like PCOS, but now most people will nod their heads if you mention it, and relate a story of someone they know who has the syndrome.

In fact, in the 1998 edition of the classic women's health bible *Our Bodies, Ourselves,* polycystic ovarian disease gets a passing reference in a paragraph relating to infertility, while fibromyalgia gets a full page devoted to diagnosis, causes, symptoms, and treatments. The next edition of *Our Bodies, Ourselves* will almost certainly devote as much space to PCOS. Friends and family will begin to nod their heads in understanding when you mention the syndrome. Hopefully, as a result, more women will go for diagnosis and treatment, instead of being thought of as hypochondriacs.

The Long Haul

Addressing the symptoms of PCOS is a long-term proposition. The good news is that alleviating and controlling many of these symptoms will ultimately create a whole new healthy you! Working with a dietitian and starting to see progress in gaining control of weight problems can be a self-esteem booster that will rocket you into tackling the other problems. And controlling weight means that many of these other problems will be less dramatic to begin with! This isn't intended to make it sound as if controlling the symptoms of PCOS will be easy— it will be a long road full of speed bumps and sharp curves. But there will also be long straight stretches that will get longer and smoother once you begin to follow the right route.

But there's the magic word—begin. In order to make progress, you need to begin taking control of PCOS instead of letting it control you.

A PERSONAL STORY

Trista

At around twenty years old, Trista went to the library and began to do some research. She was trying to find an explanation for her lack of menstrual cycles and other symptoms, such as the excess hair growth that she'd been afflicted with since her teens. Although diagnosed as simply "anovulatory," Trista was convinced there was something not quite right with her body.

Trista's determination paid off. In a small rural library, she ran across the phrase "Stein-Leventhal Syndrome." The accompanying list of symptoms described everything she was dealing with. "This is it," Trista said to herself in the library, "this is what I have." Over the next seven years she went to as many as eight doctors, none of whom would diagnose her. They had never heard of Stein-Leventhal, or if they had, they really didn't know much about it.

Trista's big break with diagnosis was when she went to a reproductive endocrinologist (R.E.). Although not quite ready to get pregnant, Trista wanted to know what was going on with her body. The R.E. did lab work and diagnosed her with PCOS. Finally. She was put on spironolactone and, because it is important not to get pregnant while on the drug, she also began taking birth control. Spironolactone has not been tested specifically for PCOS, but is often used "off-label" because it reduces the free testosterone that goes to the skin. As a result, Trista's hirsutism decreased dramatically. She took the spironolactone and birth control for a year, and then stopped both. She was ready to try getting pregnant.

Trista's doctor gave her a prescription for Clomid, an ovulation-stimulating drug, and basically said to call in thirty days. She was a bit discouraged by the hands-off approach and had been hoping for more guidance along the way. She tried ovulation detection tests, but, as the packages themselves say, they are often not effective with women with PCOS. She didn't ovulate, and she didn't get pregnant.

Then Trista moved to a more urban area and sought out a reproductive endocrinologist. Her new doctor ran several tests, including ultrasounds of her ovaries, something Trista had never had done by any of her other doctors. Her new R.E. worked with lots of PCOS patients, and Trista really felt she was on the right track. Since Clomid had not worked, her new doctor went straight to injectable fertility drugs and monitored Trista carefully, since women with PCOS can have troubles with multiple eggs.

"I was so happy to finally get a doctor who was really paying attention. And I was so thrilled to ovulate—I finally felt like a woman!" Thanks to this doctor's help, she is now the proud mother of two daughters.

Trista was so grateful to the PCOSA (www.pcosupport.org), since their site is where she found a lot of her research, that she signed on to be the president of the chapter in her region. At a recent "Women's Expo" in Minneapolis (an annual event that draws several thousand people), Trista was able to staff a booth for the organization. "We put up a huge sign listing PCOS symptoms," she said. "There was a long line at our booth. Women would look at the sign and say, 'This is it, this is what I have, I can't believe it.'"

Trista has now decided to jump to the other side of the research fence and participate in a clinical trial through the Mayo Clinic that will study the way that women with PCOS metabolize fat. The follow-up study includes five months during which Trista will receive complete handholding for diet and exercise. Who knows, perhaps a very specific diet will come of the research!

Trista has this advice for women who think they have PCOS or are struggling with the syndrome: "Get to an endocrinologist. This may sound simple, but many women think that just because OB/GYNs are focused on all things female, that is where they should go. PCOS is not a 'female problem.' It is a hormonal problem, and hormones control everything in our bodies."

CHAPTER TWO ∾

The Way It Is Meant to Be
Typical Reproductive and Endocrinological Processes

The reproductive cycle in women is a highly coordinated interaction between the physical organs of reproduction and the biochemical contributions of the endocrine system. This chapter will introduce the physical and hormonal processes involved in the reproductive scenario as it was meant to happen, so that you can better understand where PCOS contributes to breakdowns in biologic and chemical communications that interfere with pregnancy.

The Players

The key physical organs of female reproduction are the uterus, ovaries, and fallopian tubes. These three organs interact to take reproduction from conception to birth. And, in between times when they are not actually being used for their reproductive functions, they are designed to go through cycles that keep them ever-ready for their intended role. We'll discuss them individually.

The Uterus

The uterus, also commonly called the womb, is a thick-walled, muscular cavity situated deep in the pelvic region between the bladder and rectum. The uterus is where a fertilized egg matures into a fetus during the nine months of pregnancy.

The Ovaries

The ovaries are a pair of walnut-sized organs also housed within the pelvis, just behind the uterus and fallopian tubes. A woman's lifetime supply of eggs is stored in the ovaries.

The Fallopian Tubes

Although we don't tend to hear as much about them, the fallopian tubes are an important ingredient in the overall reproductive recipe. The fallopian tubes are the passageways between the ovaries and uterus that the eggs use to travel to the uterus, either to meet the male sperm, which would come in search of them, or to leave the body unfertilized. The fallopian tubes are about ten centimeters long. The outer end of each tube is funnel-shaped, ending in long fringes called fimbriae.

The tube is much more complex than a simple pipe. It has a folded lining that is covered with microscopic hair-like projections called cilia; the beating of the cilia is what pushes the egg along the tube. The tubal lining also produces a fluid that nourishes the egg during its journey to the uterus.

Each month, these organs prepare for the possibility of pregnancy in a transformation regulated by hormones.

Hormone Basics

Hormones are chemical messengers that tell cells what to do. A specific interaction occurs when a hormone traveling through the bloodstream encounters a target cell. The interaction is comparable to a lock-and-key relationship. If the hormone "key" fits the cell receptor "lock," the hormone delivers its message and the cell carries out the instruction.

A hormone circulating in your bloodstream may encounter an enzyme. An enzyme is a complex protein that causes a chemical reaction to occur. There are many hundreds of different enzymes in your body, each having a specialized function.

When an enzyme and a hormone meet, another lock-and-key opportunity arises. If the hormone-key fits into the enzyme-lock, the enzyme converts (metabolizes) the hormone into something else. The hormone may be changed into a slightly different hormone or be converted into a substance that is to be excreted from the body. Hormones need to be broken down and excreted; otherwise, they can build up and eventually cause serious health problems. Enzymatic action is a crucial part of the removal process.

Glands of the Endocrine System

The endocrine system includes nine interconnected glands that secrete hormones into the bloodstream, which then delivers these chemicals to various organs to regulate functions such as growth, sexual development, metabolism (the process by which your body utilizes the food you consume), and emotions. The endocrine glands associated with reproduction are the hypothalamus, the pituitary, the adrenal, the pancreas, and the ovaries.

The *hypothalamus,* located at the base of the brain, is the master regulator of the endocrine and nervous systems. It coordinates many bodily functions, including body temperature, metabolism, appetite, and sleep patterns. It is attached to the *pituitary gland,* a pea-sized structure at the base of the brain, which, among other functions, releases hormones that stimulate the ovaries to make estrogen. The hypothalamus provides the link between the brain and pituitary gland by producing releasing and inhibiting factors that control the pituitary gland's secretion of hormones into the blood. The *adrenal glands* contribute DHEA, and other androgenic hormones, the culprits behind some of the most frustrating symptoms that women with PCOS experience. The insulin resistance common to many women with PCOS makes the *pancreas*, which produces insulin, important in the endocrinology of PCOS. And last but not least on this list are the *ovaries*, which manufacture estrogen, progesterone, and androgens, hormones vital to successful ovulation and reproduction.

Whether the effects of hormones on the body as a whole and on the reproductive system in particular are neutral, beneficial, or damaging depends on their concentration levels in the bloodstream. The normally functioning endocrine system regulates the synthesis and secretion of hormones based on the chemical feedback systems that are especially prominent in the links between the hypothalamus and the pituitary. Negative feedback is the predominant regulating mechanism and functions much like the thermostat in your living room that regulates the furnace in the basement. When the furnace produces sufficient heat to raise the temperature above the temperature you've set in your living room, the thermostat is triggered and shuts off the furnace. When the temperature drops, the negative feedback—adequate temperature—is no longer in effect, and the furnace comes back on until the temperature is high enough to exert negative feedback again and stop the furnace from producing additional heat.

So, when your pancreas secretes insulin, the properly functioning endocrine system lets the pancreas know when the insulin level (the heat in the house) is at the level set by the hypothalamus and the pituitary (the thermostats) and to shut it off until the negative feedback (the lowering of the insulin level) drops back again, and the cycle starts over. With insulin resistance, the level is never sufficiently met because the body is not properly using the insulin that the pancreas is secreting.

The same scenario is true of the reproduction-related hormones. A lack of balance in the estrogen and androgen hormones means that the ovaries are never sure when to shut down. Excessive androgens give PCOS women the excess hair growth symptom to deal with. Improper hormone balance can mean lack of ovulation and the resulting issues with fertility that this creates.

Maintaining hormonal balance is a key job in the normally function-ing endocrine system. This role as regulator is highly evident in the menstrual history of a woman without PCOS, as you will see.

Transformative Chemistry: Puberty

Puberty marks the beginning of the physical transformation toward reproductive maturity. Body shape, hormone levels, and behavior begin to change in response to hormonal instructions. Breasts develop, pubic hair appears, bones mature, and height and weight increase; body fat ratios are known to trigger the onset of menstruation, usually between the ages of twelve and eighteen. The process of sexual matu-ration known as puberty takes about four years to complete.

Before the first menstrual period, levels of estrogen in the bloodstream fluctuate widely. The endometrium (the lining of the uterus) is affected by these initial preparatory hormonal changes until a point is reached where substantial growth of the uterine lining results.

Two years before other hormones appear in the system, generally when a girl is between the ages of nine and eleven, the hormone dehydroepiandrostenedione (DHEA) is released by an important player in the endocrine system, the adrenal glands. As a result, hair growth under the arms and in the pubic area begins. At this time, girls usually experience an increase in height and weight. This increase in body weight signals the hypothalamus to release the hormone gonadotropin-releasing hormone (GnRH). GnRH is carried to the pituitary gland through small blood vessels and stimulates the pituitary to release two hormones that instruct the ovaries to begin to produce estrogen. These are known as follicle-stimulating hormone (FSH) and luteinizing hormone (LH).

In sexually mature females, FSH (assisted by LH) acts on the follicle to stimulate it to release estrogens. LH stimulates the follicle to secrete estrogen in the first half of the menstrual cycle. A surge of LH then triggers the maturing of the egg and its release (ovulation) in the middle of the cycle. Later, LH stimulates the now-empty follicle to develop into the corpus luteum, which secretes hormones during the latter half of the menstrual cycle.

The first ovulation does not occur until six to nine months after the first menstrual period of a young girl, known as menarche.

The Nutrition Connection

The communication between the hypothalamus, pituitary gland, and ovaries is dependent on a body fat ratio of about 25 percent. It is thought that the hormone leptin, which is produced by fat cells, must achieve a certain level in the blood in order for menstruation to begin. These levels must be sustained thereafter to maintain regular menstrual cycles.

Proper nutrition is instrumental to both the onset and continuation of menstruation, and requires a balance of fat, sugars and starches (carbohydrates), and protein. Women in the 1830s typically began menstruation at an average age of seventeen, while the average age of menarche in the developed nations today is thirteen years. This shift in sexual maturity is thought to be linked to improved nutrition, although other theories regarding environmental exposure to hormones and other food additives exist as well.

Once menarche is underway, ongoing release of GnRH is necessary to maintain regular cycles. Stress and sudden changes in body weight can upset the release of this hormone. Childhood obesity may accelerate the sexual maturation process, resulting in earlier than usual menarche. During times of stress, it's not uncommon for a woman to miss a menstrual period. Women who lose significant body weight will disrupt the cycle and stop menstruating completely. And women who lose or gain weight may experience changes in their usual cycle. These changes in normal reproductive cycles are thought to be linked to the failure of the hypothalamus to release GnRH, perhaps as the body's way of ensuring that pregnancy only occurs when the mind and body of a woman are ready to support a pregnancy.

Reproductive Partners: Menstruation and Ovulation

The main events of the normal reproductive cycle are menstruation and ovulation. Monthly hormone patterns control the timing of both. Ovulation is the period when a mature egg is released, making fertilization and pregnancy possible. Menstruation is the most visible event of the cycle—when fertilization does not occur, the uterus discharges a fluid made up of blood, mucus, and endometrial cells from the uterine lining.

A Typical Menstrual Cycle

The menstrual cycle regulates fertility. Because of this cycle, the possibility of a fertilized egg reaching the uterus exists for a few days every month. For most women between roughly the ages of twelve and fifty, the menstrual cycle generally lasts between twenty-five and thirty days from start to finish, though individual variations are likely. Menstruation does not take place during the months of pregnancy or for the first months after giving birth, typically linked to the length of breastfeeding, which keeps certain hormones in circulation that are perhaps keeping the body under check because the woman is supporting one child and is not ready to bear another.

Here are the key events of the cycle, which will be described in greater detail in the pages that follow:

> *Menses, Days 0-5:* The onset of menstrual discharge, consisting of blood, endometrial cells from the uterine lining, mucus, and other fluids, is considered the beginning of the cycle and generally lasts 5-7 days.

> *Follicular Phase, Days 6-10:* The primary follicle containing the ovum develops and secretes increasing amounts of estrogen. The uterine lining begins to thicken. Follicular development is supported by low LH and FSH levels.

> *Secondary Follicular Phase, Days 11-14:* Estrogen levels are at their peak. The dominant follicle is ready for release by the ovary. The development of the uterine lining continues.

> *Ovulation, Day 15:* LH and FSH levels surge for twenty-four hours, and the egg is released from the dominant follicle. The corpus luteum (remainder of the follicle) remains in the ovary, secreting estrogen and progesterone. The uterus is ready to receive the egg.

> *Luteal Phase, Days 16-28:* The egg begins its journey along the fallopian tube to the uterus, possibly to be met by a sperm along the

way. LH and FSH levels drop as estrogen levels rise. The corpus luteum shrinks, and if fertilization does not occur, it dies, causing estrogen and progesterone levels to fall and menses to begin.

Before Ovulation

Human females are born with a lifetime's supply of eggs. At birth, the ovaries contain about a million follicles, each a collection of fluid-filled cells surrounding an immature egg. Only about 300 to 500 of these follicles will develop into mature eggs during the reproductive life span, typically between puberty and about age fifty, when the possibility of egg fertilization ends with menopause (the cessation of menstruation).

The fact that females produce eggs once a month rather than continuously is a result of the shifts in the feedback mechanisms between the ovarian and pituitary hormones during the menstrual cycle. During the fertile years, the hypothalamus, the pituitary gland, and the ovaries communicate through hormones to regulate the reproductive cycle.

During the *follicular phase* before ovulation, hormonal sequences support the growth of the follicle, which is the cellular complex that surrounds and nurtures the egg in the ovary, and signal the lining of the uterus to receive a fertilized egg. At this phase, the level of estrogen produced in the ovaries is low. In response to this low level of estrogen, GnRH secretion increases in the hypothalamus, stimulating the pituitary gland to release low levels of follicle-stimulating hormone (FSH). This is the hormone that instigates the ripening process of the follicles in the ovaries. Several days after FSH triggers continued growth in the follicle, estrogen begins to be released into the bloodstream on its way to the hypothalamus. Ten to twenty follicles will begin to develop, typically, and usually one will reach maturity, though occasionally two or more will reach this stage. The follicles also produce estrogen, and as the eggs ripen, estrogen output increases.

Small Cysts Are Normal

Small cysts on the ovaries are normal in the process of ovulation. Each month, an egg becomes encapsulated in a fluid-filled sac known as a cyst. The sac provides nourishment to the egg. These cysts appear and disappear as a normal function of the ovaries.

In order to produce estrogen, the follicles require small amounts of the luteinizing hormone (LH). LH, another pituitary hormone, stimulates the manufacture of testosterone by the ovary cells that surround the follicle, which is then transported to the inside of the follicle and converted to estrogen. This signals the uterine lining (endometrium) to thicken in preparation for the possibility of eventually nurturing a fertilized egg. This is the beginning of the second menstrual phase, *proliferation*.

By now, one follicle has become dominant and produces rapidly increasing amounts of estrogen. Some of this hormone secretion will be bound to a protein in the bloodstream known as sex-hormone-binding globulin (SHBG). During their reproductive years, women have double the concentration of SHBG when compared to men, because estrogens encourage SHBG production. Androgens, such as testosterone, suppress SHBG production.

The hormones captured by SHBG become basically inert. The production of cervical mucus begins. FSH production declines, removing support from the competing lesser follicles. Declining FSH levels also make the dominant follicle receptive to LH. When the estrogen levels are sufficient, around the middle of the cycle, and the egg approaches maturity, the follicle releases a burst of progesterone. In response, GnRH increases, signaling the pituitary to secrete large amounts of both FSH and LH. Within thirty-six hours of this surge, the now-mature follicle bursts, releasing the egg (ovulation). This is the optimum time for fertilization of the egg by male sperm.

After Ovulation

At ovulation, the follicle and the ovarian surface open over the egg. (Some women experience this as a twinge or cramp in the lower abdomen or back.) The egg is released and picked up by the finger-like tendrils of the fallopian tube. The fallopian tube itself is a highly movable muscular structure capable of precisely coordinated movement. If a woman has had sexual intercourse during this fertile time, the egg and the sperm meet in the outer half of the fallopian tube.

Under the influence of LH, the now-empty follicle is transformed in function and becomes known as the *corpus luteum*. It will take over from the hypothalamus and release both estrogen and progesterone during the proliferation phase of the cycle.

The classic "string of pearls"—a ring of cysts surrounding the outside of the ovary in most PCOS women—is thought to be the remains of follicles that, because of mixed and incorrect hormonal signals, never developed into actual eggs. As explained in Chapter One, these cysts are not the same as the "ovarian cysts" that many women also experience—the ovarian cyst is a growth inside the ovary that can enlarge and interfere with the function of the ovary. The classic cysts of PCOS are small and can even go away when PCOS is under control. It bears repeating that these cysts, often thought to be the cause of PCOS, are actually an indicator or symptom, but not a cause. And ironically, given that the syndrome is named after these cysts, many women with PCOS do not show these cysts on their ovaries at all, making PCOS a very mysterious syndrome simply by virtue of its name!

In response to the progesterone increase produced by the corpus luteum, the thickening uterine lining begins to secrete nutrients in preparation for receiving a fertilized egg. This phase can last from six to twenty days. If fertilization occurs, these nutrients will sustain a growing embryo until the placenta develops and the mother's blood supply can nourish the fetus during the rest of the pregnancy. A fertilized egg can only implant during this nourishing phase.

The Final Luteal Phase

A woman ovulates once a cycle. The egg lives twelve to twenty-four hours and then disintegrates if not fertilized. Under favorable cervical mucus conditions (cervical mucus nourishes and guides the sperm, which would otherwise die in about a half-hour or never be able to reach the egg), sperm can survive as long as five days within the body.

If the mature egg is fertilized, the corpus luteum will then provide the estrogens and progesterone necessary to sustain the pregnancy. Continued hormone production in the corpus luteum is triggered by human chorionic gonadotropin (HCG), a hormone produced by the developing placenta and chemically very similar to LH.

If the egg is not fertilized, FSH levels diminish, and LH levels also decrease as progesterone rises. The corpus luteum shrinks. Blood vessels to the thickened endometrial lining close off and stop supplying nutrients. The corpus luteum dies, as well as the unfertilized egg. The uterine lining breaks down and is shed in the process known as menstruation.

Cleansing the Uterus

The uterus is the only organ whose inner lining (endometrium) is routinely expelled and reconstructed, as happens during each menstrual cycle. The endometrium is the double-layered tissue that lines the uterus. It consists of connective tissue containing a large number of tubular-shaped glands, and its blood supply is provided by an intricate system of blood vessels. When the blood levels of the ovarian hormones fall, the supportive endometrial layer that nourishes fetal growth in pregnancy immediately exhibits signs of regression, shrink-age, and atrophy produced by the corpus luteum.

The second, inner layer of the endometrium is relatively thin and is deep within the uterus. This layer is not shed during menstruation, and it provides the foundation for a new supportive layer when the men-strual bleeding ceases and a new cycle begins. This layer does not ex-hibit significant modifications during the cycle, and seems to be less responsive to the hormonal stimuli. Its blood supply is provided by an-other vascular system, and because of this it remains intact throughout the menstrual cycle.

As the blood flow to the endometrium is reestablished, dead lining tis-sue is sloughed off and carried out of the uterus by blood. The uterus begins to produce prostaglandins, chemicals that lead to the uterine contractions that expel the accumulation of cervical mucus, vaginal se-cretions, unfertilized eggs, and endometrial tissues, as well as blood. Prostaglandins contribute to the cramping sensation many women ex-perience during menstruation. The flow lasts from four to five days for most women, and spotting may continue for another day or two. Blood lost amounts to a small fraction of the total volume of blood and does not usually impair normal physiological functions.

During the days of cleansing menstrual flow, estrogen and proges-terone levels are low, but FSH levels are sufficient to stimulate growth of the follicles waiting in the ovary. And the cycle begins anew.

What Is "Regular"?
Menstrual regularity varies from woman to woman, and sometimes varies significantly in the same woman until "irregular" may be what's considered regular! Emotional "seasons," particularly times of stress, also affect the chemical and biological events that maintain or sidetrack

menstrual regularity, as do body fat ratios and other health issues. But generally, the normal range for period cycles is considered to be between twenty-four and thirty-five days. Period cycles in which a woman does not ovulate, as is common in cases of PCOS, tend to be more irregular. Because ovulation triggers many premenstrual "warning signs," periods in the absence of ovulation tend to arrive suddenly.

Menopause

Menopause is the time when a woman has her last period, and fertility ends. "Climacteric" is another term for the transition from the reproductive to the nonreproductive years of life. The average age of menopause among women in western nations is fifty-one, though some will reach this phase during their thirties and some in their sixties. The average age of menopause has not changed much in the past few centuries.

Perimenopause is the period of gradual physical and biochemical changes that lead into menopause. The process begins when the ovaries stop releasing eggs—usually a gradual process. It can be a stop-start process that may take months or years. Sometimes it happens all at once. The typical symptoms of the menopausal transition are irregular periods and hot flashes. The average age of the onset of perimenopause is forty-seven, and the process lasts about four years. Interestingly, this four-year span is the same time span as for puberty, when reproductive capacity gets under way.

The ovaries' production of estrogen slows down during perimenopause. This phase before menopause is often characterized by irregular periods. In fact, changes such as shorter or longer periods, heavier or lighter menstrual bleeding, and varying lengths of time between periods may be a sign that menopause is near. Hormone levels fluctuate, causing various changes in body, mind, and sometimes spirit. The changes leading to menopause may seem more intense than those during puberty. All PCOS women will change from a low FSH/high estrogen phase to the high FSH/low estrogen phase of menopause.

The time after menopause is called post-menopause. Because women now experience longer life spans, modern women are usually post-menopausal for at least a third of their lives.

PCOS After Menopause

The good news is that it seems that women with PCOS begin to have more regular cycles as they approach menopause, presumably because the hormonal swings that are the trademark of PCOS lessen as a woman nears the end of her reproductive years.

The Insulin (Dis)Connection

Insulin resistance is a characteristic common among women with PCOS. This condition is defined as resistance in key organs such as muscles, liver, and fat to the glucose-sequestering effects of insulin.

Understanding the role insulin plays in PCOS means first looking at the role insulin plays in the normal metabolism of glucose. Glucose is the simple sugar that provides vital fuel to cells throughout the body. The body absorbs glucose from food in the intestines, sending it into the bloodstream for distribution throughout the body. In order to avoid starving cells overnight or oversupplying glucose right after a meal, the body strives to maintain a reliable and constant supply of energy. Excess glucose is stored in the liver and muscles as glycogen, made up of long chains of glucose. If glucose is required when it is in short supply in the bloodstream, glycogen is converted back to glucose to keep a steady blood-sugar level.

Two pancreatic hormones with opposite responsibilities take on the job of regulating and adjusting the supply of cellular fuel. *Glucagon* stimulates the liver and muscles to break down and release stored glycogen as glucose, to increase fuel from the body's stores when it's in low supply. *Insulin's* job is to store nutrients right after ingestion by reducing the concentrations of glucose, fatty acids, and amino acids in the bloodstream.

As explained in the section on basic hormone regulation, negative feedback is a prime control method in achieving chemical balance. Normal glucose regulation is another example of negative feedback. After you drink a glass of milk or eat a candy bar, glucose from the lactose (milk) or sucrose (candy) is absorbed in the intestine. The blood level of glucose then rises and stimulates endocrine cells in the pancreas to release insulin to deal with the glucose. Because insulin allows glucose to enter many cells of the body, the level in the bloodstream falls. When enough glucose has left the bloodstream, insulin is no longer secreted.

After a meal, the presence of glucose, fatty acids, and amino acids in the intestine stimulates the pancreas to release insulin into the blood, at the same time inhibiting the secretion of glucagon. As insulin levels begin to rise, body cells, especially liver, fat, and muscle cells, absorb the molecules of glucose, fatty acids, and amino acids. Thus the level of concentrations of sugars and acids in the bloodstream is kept fairly constant. However, in the case of insulin resistance, the body has a lower than usual sensitivity to insulin. The body responds by increasing insulin production in an attempt to regulate glucose levels.

Recent research indicates that insulin also plays a role in ovulation. Insulin receptors are abundant in the ovaries. In the reproductive cycle, insulin stimulates an increase in LH and sex hormone (androgen) levels, decreasing the available levels of SHBG. Because insulin blood levels can be high in women who have PCOS, androgen production in the ovaries appears to be stimulated (hypoandrogenism). At the same time, SHBG levels drop lower than usual and cannot bind with and neutralize those androgens. In the presence of overwhelming androgens, LH levels increase beyond the normal threshold and lead to poor follicle development and failure to ovulate (anovulation). The subject of insulin and PCOS is discussed further in Chapter Six, which is concerned with diet, nutrition, and weight control.

A PERSONAL STORY

Anita: In Her Own Words

I got my first period around age twelve. After the first couple, they became extremely sporadic; months would pass in between periods. I sensed something was not quite right, but was consumed with other teenage concerns and ignored it.

By the time I was fifteen, I had my third bout with mononucleosis. I thought perhaps that was the reason I was not getting a period. After recovering, I went to Planned Parenthood, had my first pelvic exam, and was afraid of what they would say. But I was quickly ushered in and out of the exam and given a supply of birth control pills. That doctor did not have the time or inclination to talk with me about my problems. I did not fully understand at the time that Planned Parenthood was not really a place to go to be diagnosed. My periods became regular but heavy and painful. I gained more weight on the pill and felt lousy. I tried to make the best of things and remained on the pill. I didn't know what else to do.

I stayed on the pill until my mid-twenties, switching prescriptions to try to find one that didn't make me feel terrible. In 1994, I'd had enough and went off the pill. My husband and I discussed at that time if we should use an alternative birth control and decided that we were open to the idea of having a baby. However, along with the end of using birth control pills also came the end of regular periods.

At first, several months would pass in between periods...then longer...over one year. Since I was open to the idea of getting pregnant, I looked through the Yellow Pages trying to figure out where to go, who to see, how to get help. My eyes fell to a fertility specialty clinic.

I saw a woman doctor at this clinic for the next couple of years. She prescribed Provera every four months or so to induce a period. She was the first doctor to ever tell me that the reason I was not menstruating was probably because I was not ovulating. This was not good news, but it was good to have some sort of answer. This doctor was the first to really listen to me and ask questions, but I still felt like she was missing something and gradually stopped seeing her.

In 2000, I went to a nurse practitioner on a completely unrelated matter. I sat on the exam table talking to her, and I felt her eyes studying me. She asked me when my last period was. I told her I couldn't really even remember, that it had been months. She asked me if I had ever heard of PCOS. I had not. She smiled at me and said, "You have a lot of reading to do." It was such a monumental moment in my life to suddenly have everything fall into place—to have a reason, even a name, for this craziness I'd been feeling about my body most of my life. I will never, ever forget this nurse practitioner, she truly changed my life and I am so grateful.

I am now thirty-one years old. I have not been using birth control of any form for over eight years, and I have never been pregnant. One other thing I have learned is that it takes a very strong marriage and a lot of love to deal with PCOS. I am grateful for my husband's support! I have not aggressively tried to get pregnant with assisted means such as fertility drugs. But now that I am aware of the options available for women with PCOS, I feel more hopeful about the prospect of starting a family.

CHAPTER THREE ∾

Key Symptoms of PCOS
Lack of Cycles, Infertility, and Weight Control

Every woman with PCOS does not experience the same set of symptoms as every other woman with the syndrome. Some women with polycystic ovaries do not exhibit any of the other symptoms of the disorder itself beyond having ovaries with the classic ring of cysts. And those who do experience many or all of the key symptoms that are signals of PCOS experience them in varying degrees of severity. What is one PCOS woman's annoyance is another PCOS woman's curse.

The discussion in this chapter revolves around the key symptoms that women who have polycystic ovarian syndrome are likely to express on some level. You may be experiencing one of these issues, or you may experience many of them.

At the top of the list are weight issues—from overweight to obese, the hormonal influence on PCOS creates the chemical imbalance in the body that distorts the way your body processes food. The good news is that while losing weight can be difficult for the PCOS patient, the benefits can be huge and immediate.

Weight Control

Nutrition, diet, and weight control are key players in the treatment and control of all the symptoms of PCOS. Diet and weight are so important, that we have devoted a whole chapter to nutrition later in this book. While a woman's diet does not cause PCOS, a poor diet and lack of good nutrition exacerbate most of its symptoms. Weight gain and actual obesity are significant issues that PCOS sufferers deal with; weight control not only helps with those problems but has proven to have positive effects on the other symptoms of the syndrome.

PCOS patients have long been considered to be high-risk individuals for coronary heart disease. This is still a topic of some debate, as reported by Bruce Jancin in the June 15, 2000, issue of *Family Practice News:* One of the more recent studies showed no increase in coronary heart disease mortality, while a Swedish study concluded that "women with PCOS are at a markedly increased risk of heart disease." What was agreed upon, however, was that "perhaps the best advice that can be provided to PCOS patients is to try to maintain a healthy body weight."

Easier said than done for women with PCOS, which is managed by managing symptoms. Being overweight makes the various symptoms of PCOS worse, but the hormonal imbalances and often the drugs used to combat them set women with PCOS up for obesity problems. Weight control is definitely possible, however, and worth pursuing. The first step is to understand what is going on.

Sometimes the drugs used in treating PCOS are partly to blame. Many classes of drugs used to treat depression, drugs for high blood pressure, antiseizure medications, steroids, and any hormone therapy have weight gain as a side effect. For women with other health problems, it is important to weigh the advantages of drug therapies against the contribution the drug plays in gaining weight and exacerbating PCOS symptoms. Of course, drugs may be the best and sometimes only solution for serious health issues, but if you are diagnosed with PCOS and are also dealing with other non-life-threatening diseases or conditions, it is worth talking with your medical team to consider other nondrug treatments for your condition. If drugs are the only course of action, you can try to offset the negative effects of weight gain by eating as healthfully as you can.

The real problem with PCOS and weight issues, however, is that at the core of the syndrome's pathology is an inability of the body to accurately use the hormone insulin. Because the body does not use the insulin it produces effectively, the pancreas keeps pumping out more (see Hyperinsulinemia for more details). This resistance to insulin makes the body turn carbohydrates to fat instead of energy. Therefore, at the same time that the PCOS sufferer is gaining weight, she is also feeling more and more fatigued. The vicious cycle continues.

As mentioned in Chapter One, PCOS weight gain is typically seen as the "apple-shape," as opposed to the "pear-shape," figure. A high hip-to-waist ratio is common and is associated with impaired glucose and insulin metabolism. Anecdotal evidence, according to the PCOS support group Polycystic Ovarian Syndrome Association (www.pcosupport.org), seems to indicate that women with PCOS do not have as much success with the standard low-fat diet as women who aren't affected. Women with PCOS typically find more success by both reducing total carbohydrate intake and picking different carbohydrates to eat. Replacing refined carbohydrates with whole grains, fruits, and vegetables not only helps reduce insulin response but also increases the daily intake of essential micronutrients, such as the beneficial group known as antioxidants.

Herein lies the glucose/insulin PCOS/diabetes connection. To the person who is attempting to control diabetes, checking blood sugar levels at least daily, and usually several times a day, is almost as natural as breathing. Because the body afflicted with diabetes is unable to deal with insulin in the way it was designed to, the body is also unable to effectively regulate its own blood sugar. Therefore, diabetics have to help their bodies do this by eating in a prescribed manner, controlling the glucose level of their blood. It's like the difference between an automatic shift and a manual shift car—in one, the automatic transmission is designed to control the engine speed for you; in the other, you need to use the clutch and the gas in concert to control the engine speed yourself.

This means that as a woman with PCOS, like the person with diabetes, you need to get behind the controls to regulate your blood-sugar levels. While keeping in mind that so far nothing is certain when it comes to PCOS, it appears that the first dietary challenge the PCOS patient faces is regulating carbohydrate intake. This will help to regulate blood-sugar levels, which can become low since the pancreas is being told inaccurately to pump out more insulin than is really necessary.

The human body stores a considerable amount of energy as fat. Although the 90s saw Americans going through a low-fat frenzy, this rainy day fat reserve is not obtained only by eating foods that contain fat. To maintain a good body weight, you need to combine the right amount of carbohydrates, protein, and fat, and further regulate it with an exercise regimen appropriate to weight loss, first, and then to weight control.

The complexity of the best diet for a PCOS patient makes it clear how important it is for the woman with PCOS to work with a registered dietitian, in order to build the most workable eating plan—which is discussed in further detail in Chapter Six. However, simply put, weight loss helps to return hormones to normal levels, so the importance of weight control for PCOS patients cannot be emphasized too much.

There are, of course, more drastic measures that can be taken for the severely overweight woman who has tried everything to lose weight and cannot succeed. Liposuction is a commonly known procedure that simply sucks the fat out from under the skin around the hip and thigh areas. Since women with PCOS experience the "apple shape" in weight gain, this is probably not a useful course of treatment. The most drastic measures include jaw wiring, in which the jaw is literally wired partially shut so that only liquids can pass through. Once you reach your target weight through this forced dieting plan, the jaw is unwired—and quite often the weight returns. Also drastic and more commonly discussed in the media of late, is the dieting technique known as stomach stapling. Basically, a portion of the stomach is stapled off, making it smaller and unable to contain as much. The person with the stapled stomach feels full faster and so isn't able to eat as much. This is a really extreme weight control measure and should only be considered as a very last resort. Also, it should be considered that a lot of women with PCOS do not overeat, but still gain weight because PCOS is working on the metabolic level—what they do eat is just not being processed normally by their bodies.

While this is a significant issue for a large percentage of women with PCOS, not all experience weight problems. In fact, the statistics for obesity in women with PCOS almost mirror the obesity statistics for women as a whole. However, anecdotal evidence finds that women with PCOS gain weight more easily and find it more difficult to lose weight. It's clear that early diagnosis can be very helpful in controlling weight from the start.

You need to be very careful in managing weight. Don't get caught up in crash diets and other "too good to be true" weight control measures. They are unhealthy, period. If a diet says you can lose a hundred pounds in two months, say no thanks. Losing weight faster than a couple of pounds a week typically causes loss of muscle mass as well. This means that if you diet and lose weight in a healthy way, you will need almost a year to lose one hundred pounds! In Chapter Six, we will offer more specifics about good nutrition, weight control, and the importance of understanding good dieting practices.

The extreme end of the weight control scale is eating disorders such as anorexia and bulimia. Anorexia nervosa is a debilitating form of starvation that can lead to death. Bulimia nervosa is an eating disorder characterized by binging on food then purging the system of it by many possible means, including self-induced vomiting, diuretics, laxatives, and even excessive exercise. Many PCOS women are driven to these life-threatening disorders in their desperate attempt to control their weight, since women with PCOS often gain weight despite the fact that they are not eating much at all.

If you are one of the millions of women who have developed eating disorders in the attempt to deal with weight issues, you need to get help immediately. If you think anyone you know may be anorectic or bulimic, urge her to seek help. There are support groups and clinics across the country that can help women with eating disorders get back on track. Both anorexia and bulimia can cause irreversible damage to the body. The good news is that these disorders can be overcome.

Amenorrhea and Oligomenorrhea
Words with the suffix "-menorrhea" relate to your monthly periods. Painful periods are known as "dysmenorrhea;" irregular periods are called "oligomenorrhea;" the complete absence of periods is called

"amenorrhea;" and periods with heavy flow use a little variation on the suffix and are called "menorrhagia." A woman with PCOS can experience all of these menstrual dysfunctions, although painful periods are perhaps the least common of the menstrual-related symptoms found in PCOS patients.

The first signs of polycystic ovarian syndrome often show up when a young woman is starting her menstrual cycle. It is quite common for any young girl's first few periods to be irregular as her hormones themselves regulate, and in turn regulate her menstrual cycle. However, once menstruation has started in a teen or preteen, it is abnormal for the periods to then disappear altogether.

If you are a teenager reading this book and you started your period a while ago but haven't had one in a few months or more, do not ignore this absence of periods. Talk with a parent and your doctor, so you can begin to get regular again. And good for you for starting so young to take control of your own health!

Chances are more likely that you are a mother of a daughter who is experiencing lack of regularity with her periods, or you experienced this irregularity yourself as a young girl and it was dismissed as normal adjustment. It is within the range of normal to miss periods for a short number of months, but within the course of a year or so your body should become adjusted to this new activity it has to perform, and you should move into a regular cycle. That cycle is not the same for every woman, so you may have your own "irregularities" within that cycle— perhaps your period comes every twenty-one days instead of twenty-eight. Perhaps it is "normal" for you to skip a cycle every eight months. Whatever the case, establishing what is normal for you is the important thing. You will want to keep track of your cycles as you begin to see success in your combating of PCOS, and your cycles start to respond.

The absence of periods in PCOS patients comes from the malfunctioning of the body's hormones. Insulin resistance, common with PCOS, causes the pancreas to produce more insulin, and the chain of events is in place. PCOS causes higher than normal levels of estrogen and androgen. These high levels are sustained instead of fluctuating; it takes fluctuating hormones to create monthly periods. Basically, the wrong hormone signals give the pituitary gland the wrong message, and ovulation—and ultimately the menstruation cycle—never begins.

The increased insulin production tells other hormones to do or not do things that they normally should or shouldn't do, including signaling the body to produce more male hormones. Male hormones, as you might guess, are not the kind that tell the body to start shedding the lining of the uterus and producing a monthly period. So here we are back at the absence or irregularity of the menstrual cycle.

This excess of male hormones also results in other annoying symptoms, such as hair growth in areas that women don't usually deal with. These "secondary symptoms" are explained in the next chapter.

PCOS is just one of many disorders or problems that can cause menstrual irregularities, such as:

- A tumor on the adrenal gland can cause the gland to malfunction and produce abnormally high amounts of androgens.

- Hyperthyroidism causes the thyroid to produce excessive amounts of thyroid hormone.

- Hypothyroidism, the complete opposite of hyperthyroidism, slows down the protein that binds estrogen and testosterone and makes it usable and not free-floating.

- Hyperprolactinemia is a condition in which the pituary gland overproduces the hormone prolactin, which is the stimulant for breast milk production, which in turn suppresses ovulation.

These are just a few of the possible causes of amenorrhea. The good news is that hormonal causes can usually be detected through blood tests, although there still may be some frustrating investigative work to follow once a hormonal disruption is recognized.

Obesity is another cause of lack of periods. Although obesity itself isn't tested through the blood, obesity causes hormonal imbalances, so blood work can give indications of what's going on in the body that may be caused by obesity.

The levels of estrogen and testosterone floating around in your body at any given moment are carefully regulated by a protein called sex-hormone-binding globulin (SHBG). This protein is produced by the liver, which is very good at its job. However, fat also produces the female hormone estrogen, and so being overweight causes an excess amount of estrogen, often more than your liver's natural production of SHBG can keep up with. Imbalanced hormones mean irregular periods.

If it isn't frustrating enough that being overweight can result in amenorrhea, it gets even more frustrating to learn that it is also caused by the complete opposite—being too thin. The female body is designed to have periods only when a certain body fat ratio is reached, so extremely low body fat, like that seen in most competitive athletes, can be the underlying cause of amenorrhea. If you are an athlete in training, don't ignore your irregular cycle. If you are in training for competition, it may be unlikely that you will be willing to change your training routine enough to trigger your menstrual cycle. However, if you are an athlete who is simply into fitness and you have stopped having periods, you should seriously consider your overall health and work with a trainer and doctor to alter your fitness training—you may be surprised how little alteration it takes to have normal periods.

Hyperinsulinemia

Jennifer Couzin wrote in *Newsweek*, "Many PCOS women do not respond properly to insulin; when they eat a meal, the insulin released by the pancreas isn't enough to move glucose into the cells the way it's supposed to, so the body keeps pumping out more hormone."

As we saw in Chapter Two, which discusses the way the body is supposed to work when all systems are functioning normally, the body is made up of an astounding number of checks and balances that keep blood glucose levels at the exact right balance before, during, and after every meal. When things are not functioning properly, the body can experience either hypoglycemia (an excess of insulin, resulting in low blood-sugar levels that disrupt brain function and can cause unconsciousness) or hyperglycemia (failure to produce enough insulin to regulate blood sugar, resulting in dangerously high glucose levels that disrupt brain function, causing disorientation).

Insulin is a hormone that your body makes in the pancreas. It is the vehicle by which your body's cells use glucose. When you eat food, the glucose level in your body rises (how much it rises depends on the kind of food you eat), and your body's cells use that glucose. When glucose levels begin to fall, the body begins to use a stored glucose that is sitting in the liver and muscles in the form of glycogen. The glycogen, which is basically a long chain of glucose, has to break down again into glucose. An inefficient process at best, but an important one. Our brain functions almost exclusively on glucose. Now you can see why insulin and glucose levels are so important.

Hyperinsulinemia is the name of the condition that occurs when there is a high level of insulin in your blood. Women with PCOS often experience insulin resistance—the cells in the body become resistant to insulin. So the pancreas, thinking that the message isn't getting through, makes more insulin. The cycle continues until the pancreas gets a little exhausted and is no longer able to maintain the higher levels of insulin production; the body then becomes intolerant to all the glucose.

It becomes evident why insulin levels need to be regulated in order to control the serious side effects that occur as a result of high or low blood sugar.

Hot Flashes

The symptom known as the "hot flash" commonly exhibits itself in several ways: rapid heart beat, rise in temperature, clammy palms, and sweating are typically experienced either individually or all at once. Each woman has her own pattern of frequency, and the good news is that this pattern, with careful attention, allows you to anticipate and regulate your hot flashes a little, to attempt to offset major discomfort.

Hot flashes are most commonly associated with menopause. The normal functions of the pituitary gland and the hypothalamus, which regulates body temperature, are interrupted by the lessening presence of estrogen during menopause. Since hot flashes are caused by fluctuating hormones, whatever the underlying cause of the hormone disturbance, hot flashes can be the result. Which means, with the understanding that PCOS is an endocrine disorder, it makes sense that women with PCOS can experience hot flashes. If you are over the age of forty-five and have had somewhat regular periods throughout your life, even if you have PCOS your hot flashes may be due to premenopausal symptoms.

But if you are in your early to mid-thirties, the average age of the woman who has recently been diagnosed with PCOS, you probably are not going into menopause. Working with your doctor to get your hormonal imbalances balanced is the first step. From there, you will probably need to control hot flashes by treating the symptom itself.

If blood work shows that your body is having issues with hormone control, your doctor may prescribe drug therapies. Chances are in that case you are having many other symptoms besides hot flashes, and your need to take care of those will be greater than the need to control hot flashes—and the hot flashes may well disappear in the process. The hot flashes themselves are not a health problem, and they certainly aren't life-threatening, but they can be uncomfortable and embarrassing since you have little control over when they are going to occur.

Until the hormones are balanced, the symptom is still there to deal with. Chapter Nine, "Alternative Approaches for Managing PCOS," offers some useful tips for hot flashes, but some basic advice is:

- Dress in layers so you can control your own body temperature from the exterior as you go in and out of doors, go into different rooms that have different temperatures, or experience different situations in which you may become flushed.

- Avoid alcohol and other food and drink that cause flushing.

- Nicotine decreases circulation, so if you are a smoker, here is yet another reason to stop!

Infertility
Fertility decreases with age; it's a simple fact. A woman in her thirties is producing fewer eggs than she was when she was in her twenties. If

she is seeking to conceive, she needs to consider the fact that she may not be ovulating at every cycle. The age factor comes into play especially with PCOS women because, while all the possibilities are being investigated, it can be quite a long time before their actual problem is diagnosed. Then the process of controlling PCOS begins, which takes some time as well. The clock, as they say, is ticking.

Women often come to a diagnosis of PCOS via the fertility clinic. Again, a diagnosis is postponed because, as with the normal process of settling into your menstrual cycle, it can often take a few months from the time a woman and her partner decide to work at getting pregnant to the time when pregnancy actually happens, even under the best of circumstances. Sometimes residual protection from birth control needs to work through the system, and sometimes the couple takes time to figure out when the woman is ovulating—many things need to be in place for pregnancy to actually occur.

Once a couple has taken a while to attempt pregnancy on their own and it's not working, many other steps can still come before PCOS becomes a suspicion. Male sperm count and other potential problems with the male partner are considered. A woman may spend months attempting to lose weight, since being overweight is a known factor in problems with getting pregnant.

Of course, with the PCOS woman, as we have seen, the biggest fertility issue revolves around having a regular cycle. No cycle means no ovulation—you can't get pregnant without an egg in position to be fertilized.

If you are having a menstrual cycle—regular or not—and are not getting pregnant, then both you and your partner will want to begin being examined for fertility. A sample of his sperm will be tested for quantity and for percentage of "normal sperm"—that is, the number of sperm in the sample that are healthy enough and strong enough to swim the distance to meet the egg. A good diet without excessive caffeine, alcohol, and/or nicotine is recommended for the production of healthy sperm.

Women can expect several factors to be checked. As we discussed, as long as a menstrual cycle is happening, it then needs to be confirmed that actual ovulation is taking place. Follicle growth viewed via ultrasound, and blood work showing whether or not progesterone is rising are two ways to determine ovulatory status.

If you are in fact ovulating, then the other components of the reproductive system need to be checked, including the condition of the uterus to accept the fertilized egg and the functioning of the fallopian tubes.

Sexually transmitted diseases and infections can cause damage to the reproductive organs that may impede the ease with which a woman can become pregnant.

But don't despair! Many of the issues that can be discovered can also be fixed. And scientific breakthroughs in the high-stakes, high-incidence game of infertility are happening all the time. If your diagnosis is PCOS, then your "repair work" becomes a multi-step process, so you can't spend too much time in a funk—you have work to do! Depression can add to difficulty of getting pregnant as well as take the pleasure or even the desire out of the natural sexual activity that needs to happen before you can get pregnant in the first place. So cheer up, you have a diagnosis and can now start turning it around.

With the PCOS diagnosis, the woman seeking to get pregnant will most likely need to work on several primary symptoms at once. We'll go into this process in more detail in the chapter on fertility, but the intertwining symptoms that need to be addressed are:

- The menstrual cycle needs to be regulated.

- Obesity or even minor weight problems need to be addressed.

- Underweight women need to increase their body fat in order to stimulate menstruation.

- Insulin levels need to be regulated to ensure proper balance of male and female hormones.

- Blood-sugar levels—controlled by diet and insulin—need to be regulated, since otherwise they can cause lack of sex drive and other side effects that suppress sexual desire.

All women with PCOS can be encouraged by numerous stories of women who have become pregnant and had healthy children despite their PCOS diagnosis. Some PCOS patients have children after much hard work attacking symptoms, and some get pregnant without much more difficulty than they might have had without a PCOS diagnosis.

Don't forget that many factors can contribute to fertility problems. And some of the most important things you can do for PCOS symptoms— such as eating well and getting plenty of exercise—are also good for anyone trying to become pregnant, as well as for the ease of your pregnancy and the health of your baby.

A discussion of infertility cannot end without mentioning the important effect of stress on fertility. High stress level is a known factor in impeding conception—and the catch-22 is, of course, that infertility can itself cause stress. For women trying to deal with the frustrating symptoms of PCOS—weight gain, excess hair, hot flashes—the stress level can be an added issue affecting fertility.

Cysts on Ovaries

Polycystic ovarian syndrome—many cysts on the ovaries. The math seems simple, but as is typical with PCOS, it is not that straightforward! Yes, the classic sign of PCOS is the ultrasound that shows an ovary covered with cysts. These cysts are thought to be caused by eggs that never leave the ovary because of the abnormal cycling experienced by the woman with PCOS. The egg follicles collect around the border of the ovary in a pattern commonly referred to as a "string of pearls."

However, PCOS patients do not always have the classic cysts on the ovaries. They may have many other symptoms among the collection common for PCOS patients, but not the cysts.

It is important to note that the cysts that are present in many PCOS patients are not the same kind as those referred to as "ovarian cysts." Ovarian cysts are found in the interior of the ovary, and they are usually larger than the cysts associated with PCOS. They also can be quite painful if they rupture or rotate, whereas the ring of cysts classic to PCOS are not typically noticed at all by the woman who has them.

Cysts that are quite numerous and prominent along the edge of the ovary have been implicated in a painful condition in which the ovary twists and the cysts obstruct the ovary from turning back. This is rare and is treated with a laparoscopic procedure in which the ovary is physically turned back.

The cysts of polycystic ovaries are not typically removed. The process would be far too complicated if there are many of them, and the concern is also that too much of the ovary would also be removed. If you are experiencing difficulty getting pregnant, the cysts may be interfering with the movement of eggs in the ovary, and this is something to investigate. However, removal of the ring of cysts is not common and usually not recommended.

Where to Go from Here

Each woman with PCOS needs to work with her doctor to attack the symptoms she is experiencing. The underlying endocrinological symptoms will of course be a key target, since they are responsible for many of the other symptoms. However, rest assured, as you are working on regulating hormones, you don't need to just ignore the less systemic symptoms of PCOS.

In the next chapter we will outline many of the secondary symptoms that women often experience along with the key symptoms of polycystic ovarian syndrome. You and your doctor will decide which symptoms require visits with specialists, which symptoms will lessen as other symptoms are dealt with, and which symptoms can be treated with alternative therapies and topical treatments.

It is important that you feel you are tackling the symptoms that are of the most concern to you, however primary or secondary they are. Yes, you surely want your body's hormones balanced and your cholesterol at healthy levels. But if worry over excess hair growth is keeping you awake at night and causing you to avoid having a social life, that is a symptom you should probably consider as important as the key medical symptoms that PCOS will require you to attend to. Don't underestimate the importance of your individual experience with this syndrome; you want your primary care doctor and your medical team treating you, not the syndrome.

A PERSONAL STORY

Sheila

Sheila's story is really about her daughter, Megan, but Sheila has been a key driver in the search for the source of her daughter's increasing problems.

Unlike many women ultimately diagnosed with PCOS, Megan's periods had always been regular, but they were heavy and accompanied by a considerable amount of pain and discomfort. By the time Megan headed off to college, her doctor suggested she go on the pill, assuming that it might help the problems with her periods and a significant issue with acne.

Megan stayed on the pill for a while, but the summer of her sophomore year she went off. As a college athlete, Megan trained very hard. But she was experiencing extraordinary fatigue. She went back on the pill, but felt much worse. She now was skipping periods and didn't have a cycle for over six months.

During her junior year, she took off for France for a semester abroad. While she was there, she wrote to her mother that she was gaining weight and experiencing skin problems, not just on her face but on other parts of her body.

"I didn't pay too much attention at the time," Sheila said. "Cheese, croissants, who's not going to gain weight in France?" Sheila and her husband were scheduled to visit. "When I saw her, I almost fell over backwards." In just a few short months, Megan had gained not just a little weight, but twenty-five pounds. She had terrible acne, and her skin was darkened in places like her upper lip. Megan was now going on almost a year without having a period. Megan had had a health screening before she left for France, and the only significant thing that had shown up was high cholesterol. They assumed she had inherited that from her father, who also had extremely high cholesterol. But now Sheila "knew there was something way off." She tried to hide her shock at her daughter's appearance, and simply recommended that Megan start to eat on a diabetic-like diet.

A self-described "bulldog about her kids" and a researcher at heart, Sheila took to the Internet. She found a reference to PCOS. She talked with Megan's doctor and lined up a series of tests, from blood work to ultrasounds, for Megan to take over her break. Megan stepped off the plane on a Sunday and on Monday went to get her tests done.

While their nurse practitioner agreed there was a high probability that PCOS was the culprit, they wanted to rule out all other factors. Then the ultrasound came back, and there in black and white was the classic ring of cysts. They were recommended to an endocrinologist at the Lahey Clinic, near Boston.

The endocrinologist started Megan on Glucophage, a drug that improves the body's response to insulin. Within a month, she had her first period in quite a while. She headed back to school, started training hard again, and then had no more periods. The doctor upped her Glucophage dose, but Megan got a bit sick from it, so they dropped it back.

Her periods reappeared, but Sheila and Megan really didn't feel that there had been much of a resolution. She is now a senior in college and, after dealing with this for over a year and a half, Megan has made some progress. Her weight is back within ten pounds of what her normal weight seems to be. And her cholesterol is down to a more normal level.

"Since my husband has always had genetically high cholesterol, we eat very healthfully anyway," Sheila says. We did a joint approach over the summer. It's harder at school, Megan's not a fanatic, but she chooses to eat healthfully for the most part too. No one is going to be harmed by eating healthfully."

Not only is Megan's PCOS under control, but she has probably gained a lot by recognizing the problem at such a young age. By the time she is ready, if she chooses to have children, she will be way ahead of the fertility game. She has instituted a healthful eating style, one of the hardest changes for anyone who is trying to lose weight for any reason.

Besides her own determination about her kids and her willingness to dig in and seek things out, Sheila attributes much of their success to the enlightened medical professionals that they have encountered.

But something else nags at Sheila. Her sister-in-law died of the complications of anorexia. She was always overweight, and she always desperately wanted to have children but never could get pregnant. Although she will never know for sure, after researching PCOS and getting into the details, Sheila looks back and sees the signs all over her sister-in-law. She would like to save other women from her sister-in-law's fate.

"This thing is so hard to deal with. Your friends and family have never heard of it—you say what your daughter has and people's eyes glaze over." Sheila finds that when she relates it to diabetes, she gets more understanding.

"It's like multiple sclerosis symptoms in the '50s," she says. "A woman went to the doctor and said she was having dizzy spells, and she was told to go home and take a nap." Sheila would like to see PCOS more out in the open so that people with the symptoms will go find out what they can do to get their bodies functioning normally.

CHAPTER FOUR ∾

Secondary Symptoms
Hair Growth, Hair Loss, Acne, and Other Aggravations

While primary symptoms of PCOS are things that impair your overall health, secondary symptoms can be the most prominent, noticeable, annoying, and/or embarrassing ones of all. Secondary symptoms are often the result of the root causes of the primary symptoms—once these causes are isolated and treated, the secondary symptoms often subside all on their own.

That is good news, but the frustration comes when you are working on diagnosing and treating the primary symptoms—hormonal imbalances, weight problems, and so on—and the secondary symptoms rage on. The best thing to do is to treat your secondary problems by dealing with each symptom. We will discuss some of the possible treatments below; also be sure to check the chapter on alternative therapies for more ideas on dealing with these annoying issues.

The important thing is not to become so focused on the secondary symptoms that you don't take the time and energy to work on alleviating the primary symptoms and root causes of PCOS. That is how you will see long-term relief from the secondary symptoms as well, so it is important to tackle the basics. In the meantime, the non-health-threatening symptoms such as hair gain, hair loss, and acne can be kept at bay. No one is going to say it is an easy task, but once you have some ideas of things you can do, you can work them into your daily habits and feel that you are taking control of the things you can.

Don't hesitate to talk with your doctor about any of the secondary symptoms you may be having. Your doctor can give you referrals to specialists such as dermatologists and counselors who can help you work through all of these intertwining pieces of the puzzle that PCOS has presented you with.

Hirsutism

Pronounced "her-se-tism," this symptom of PCOS is among the most frustrating of all. While not life-threatening, dark hair growth ranks high up there on the visibility scale, next to excess weight. But whereas many people are overweight in varying degrees, with or without PCOS, therefore making that issue a less generally noticeable one, facial hair in enough quantity to require shaving can really put a woman over the top.

Dark facial hair and heavy hair growth on the upper thighs, forearms, and chest are the territory of men. The female body is not designed to have a five o'clock shadow and require daily face shaving. For the women with PCOS who experience severe hirsutism, it can be the bane of their existence. For teenagers whose PCOS symptoms rise as they approach puberty, the teasing and ostracism that their classmates and peers subject them to can be a severe early blow to self-esteem.

Sometimes things are less difficult to deal with if we face them head-on and understand what is happening. Just what is going on with the woman whose PCOS leads to excess hair growth?

Beards, moustaches, and other hair growth patterns associated with men are dictated by the male hormones. As we saw in Chapter Two, women have male hormones in their bodies, and men have female hormones as well. Typically, the genetic makeup of the cells that determines the different sexes regulates the amount of hormones according to sex. Men's bodies release the appropriate amount of male hormones and fewer female hormones, and vice versa.

In the body of the woman with PCOS, things aren't moving along quite as they were designed to do. Hormone imbalances relate to problems with the thyroid, the pituitary gland, the adrenal glands, and other hormone-producing parts of the endocrine system. With PCOS, as we have learned, often the inability of the woman's body to regulate the hormone insulin plays a large part in the lack of normal regulation of other hormones, including the sex hormones estrogen and testosterone.

A common scenario with women with PCOS is the overproduction of the male hormones known collectively as androgens. The hair follicles in the skin contain androgen receptors, which respond to the increase of androgens in the system. The fact that these hair follicles are especially sensitive to androgens explains why hair-growth patterns common to men are experienced by women with PCOS.

Of course, the key is to work with your medical team to treat the underlying cause of your PCOS, which, in turn, will eventually regulate the affected parts of your endocrine system. But in the meantime, you will be anxious to deal with the hair growth that you are experiencing every day.

Many women go the traditional routes of shaving with razors and plucking with tweezers. Keep in mind that these methods actually disturb the hair follicle itself, which in some cases can make matters worse.

Creams and waxes designed to remove hair can provide increased success and longer results. If your hair growth is not dramatic, perhaps just lightening the hair will work. Creams and waxes can irritate skin sensitivities, so don't use these products for the first time on your whole face. Try a small patch of hair first in a place that is typically hidden. Skin sensitivities can take twenty-four to forty-eight hours to show up, so give it a couple days before treating more visible parts of your body. And keep in mind that skin sensitivities can arise at any time; just because you've used a product successfully for a month, that does not mean that it will never cause irritation. Always be watchful for signs that your skin is becoming sensitive to a product, and be prepared to stop using it.

There are also longer-term hair removal treatments such as laser removal and electrolysis. These are not permanent but can be very effective and help you deal with this annoying issue without having to do something about it every day. If you are an extremely busy, active person, you may get more out of the longer-term route of laser treatments and electrolysis—if you can afford these methods, they will save you time.

If you never get in a bathing suit, then excess hair on your thighs is something only you—and anyone you choose—will know about. If you are headed to that dream vacation with a new partner, perhaps the expense of a more dramatic treatment is worth it, on a case-by-case basis. Try the different possibilities and see which ones work best for you. Again, don't try something new out of the blue, the day before you board the plane to Tahiti. Try a new method a month or two before the dream vacation is scheduled, and see how you react. You may have to try something else, so give yourself the time to do that.

If you feel comfortable with your hairdresser, don't be afraid to ask for her or his suggestions—these professionals have access to knowledge about this kind of thing that the everyday person does not. The salon you go to may even offer some treatments that you didn't realize were available.

Only you can decide the balance of time, money, and effectiveness that fits your needs. If you have been dealing with PCOS for a while, you are probably already working your way through the maze of options for hirsutism, although some women with PCOS don't experience hair growth problems at all. And as you begin to gain control of PCOS, you will find the need for any of the treatments will lessen.

Alopecia (Hair Loss)

If excess hair growth isn't enough to deal with, the woman with PCOS may also experience alopecia androgenetica, the female version of male-pattern baldness. So while you are experiencing hair growth on the rest of your body, the hair on your head—the place where you would prob-ably never complain about excess hair—is starting to thin dramatically. A classic example of what a roller-coaster ride having PCOS is!

As with hirsutism and acne, the key to reversing this process is balancing the hormones throughout your body. Birth-control pills have been impli-cated in hair thinning, but sometimes just changing the brand of pill can help, or just waiting for your hormones to balance.

In the meantime, scalp massages and stimulating shampoos can help. If you are not accustomed to being especially particular with your hair, now is the time to start. Stop buying your hair products in the local dis-count warehouse, and start working with your hairdresser to find some especially healthful products for your hair. Blow-drying or using a curling iron on your hair every day can be damaging—you don't need to add these physical methods to the hormonal ones that are already taking a toll on your hair's growth. See the chapter on alternative treatments for other things you can do to help give your hair the best possible care and make it shine and seem fuller.

Acne
The PCOS side effect of acne is another issue that is again not life-threatening but extremely annoying. You thought that by the time you were an adult, this would all be over, right? Like hair growth and weight issues, adult acne is another symptom that can be a heavy blow to a woman's self-esteem.

Acne is yet another symptom of PCOS that is related to the hormone imbalance. Sebaceous glands in the skin produce oil and are known to be sensitive to testosterone. The overabundance of this male hormone commonly found in women with PCOS often causes the sebaceous glands to overreact, blocking the pores and causing more acne than the average adult woman tends to experience. And PCOS patients often experience acne not only on their faces—acne more classic to puberty—but on the back, chest, and shoulders.

While you are working on the endocrine system side of things, you will also be attacking symptoms, like those in this chapter, individually. The double good news is that, again, not all women with PCOS have difficulty with acne, and for those who do, once the hormone imbalances start to get under control, the acne will subside.

Other Skin Issues
Skin tags and dark patches of skin (technically known as acanthosis nigricans) are also common occurrences for women with PCOS.

Miscarriage

Fertility issues fall under the previous chapter on "key symptoms" and are significant enough to women with PCOS to warrant their own chapter later in the book. However, once a woman with PCOS is pregnant, she may have a higher than normal risk of miscarriage, according to some statistics.

Miscarriage within the first twelve weeks of pregnancy is as high as 15 percent on average for women across the board. With the extra issues that women with PCOS are faced with—heightened levels of LH (luteinizing hormone), difficulties maintaining a nutritional and hormonal balance, weight issues, and increased stress—it makes some practical sense that women with PCOS would have a higher rate of miscarriage. The specific reason for the increased risk is not known, and it is likely that the reasons would be different for each woman—as different as the individual experiences with PCOS itself.

Sleep Issues

The hormonal fluctuations underlying PCOS can lead to difficulty getting a full night's restful sleep. Although PCOS symptoms as a rule aren't associated with extreme pain, there are symptoms that may cause some discomfort, perhaps even enough to interrupt your sleep. Drugs you are taking for PCOS symptoms can contribute to or even cause insomnia.

Of course, the biggest factor contributing to the sleep problems of women with PCOS is probably that of the worry and anxiety that the various symptoms produce. Women whose main problem is weight gain may be constantly hashing through the question of why their exercise program combined with subsisting on almost nothing more than air still does not help them shed the pounds. Women with hirsutism, alopecia, acne, and other more prominent symptoms may lie awake wondering if the man they found attractive at the market noticed their facial hair or could get beyond acne to their wonderful personality. The woman who is trying to get pregnant is a prime candidate for sleep problems. The thought processes brought on by PCOS can be endless.

Again, discuss this with your doctor. PCOS may have nothing to do with your sleeplessness; you need to find out what is causing it. Don't start right off taking medication to help you sleep; there are dozens of simple things you can do to enhance your night's sleep that are inexpensive and don't require drugs. Many are discussed in further detail in the chapter on alternative treatments, but here are some basic things to think about:

> Start by giving your bedroom an in-depth analysis. Is the bed comfortable and high-quality? Or is it the same bed you've been sleeping on for twenty years? Is the bedroom clutter-free? Are there electronic appliances in the bedroom, such as a television or computer? If the computer has to be in the bedroom, be sure to turn it off completely at night, and even unplug it to get rid of all those low hums and glowing lights. If you insist on having a television on to fall asleep by, be sure to set the sleep timer. Perhaps using the sleep timer on your radio to play low, soft music for an hour will help put you to sleep in the first place. Is the room a soothing color? If it's on the street side of your house and your street is busy all hours of the night, can you make another room your bedroom?

> Lavender and other herbs and oils are known to be soothing and sleep-enhancing. Use sachets near your bed, or keep a spritzer of a soothing essential oil in the bedroom.

> Get the dog or cat (or dogs/cats!) off the bed. Rover can start out snuggling cozily at your feet, but somewhere in the wee

hours of the morning he shoves his way into more than half the bed—even ten-pound cats can take up an amazing amount of room. If you get him a soft bed that he really likes and put it near yours, he can be content to be protecting you without stealing your covers.

Good sleep is essential to good health and to managing chronic health issues such as PCOS. Sleeplessness can be one of the easiest things to cure, but it definitely shouldn't be ignored.

Fatigue

Given the previous discussions about sleep problems with PCOS, it's no wonder fatigue is also an issue. But fatigue can be caused by a number of other things besides sleepless nights. If you are getting a pretty good night's sleep, then you need to address the other possibilities for fatigue. This is something you should definitely talk with your doctor about.

The hormonal imbalances you are experiencing when you have PCOS can be a major factor in fatigue. The body is designed to have functions in sync; when it is not operating as planned, fatigue is a major issue.

If you are taking any medications to combat PCOS symptoms, these can often be implicated in fatigue issues. Again, mention your fatigue to your doctor, find out if fatigue is one of the side effects of any of your medication, and then discuss the options for other drugs.

Your pharmacist can also assist you in learning about the drugs you are taking. Pharmacies these days are becoming very consumer-education oriented, providing the patient with extensive literature regarding their medications. Don't ignore this information. Although you will have discussed it with your doctor when you both agreed that going on the drug was a good idea, the information provided through the pharmacy often includes additional facts about the drug that are good to know. Keep these printouts in a file for future reference.

Besides sleeplessness and drugs, there are other things that can contribute to fatigue. The constant mental activity that occurs when something like PCOS is on your mind can itself be fatiguing.

And don't forget, maybe the fatigue is not directly related to PCOS. Polycystic ovarian syndrome has so many symptoms that it is often thought to be responsible for everything that the PCOS patient is experiencing! What with the long diagnosis process and the ongoing treatment for your PCOS symptoms, you probably think you have gone to the doctor so much more than the average person that everything about you has been checked and rechecked. But it's still important to have regular annual physicals, gynecological exams, mammograms, colon cancer checks, and all the other procedures that are pertinent for your age group. That way you can begin to rule out certain possibilities, such as anemia, in the search for the source of your fatigue.

Irritability and Mood Swings
Even doctors would probably get irritable with having to spend as much time on examinations, blood work, and detailed case histories as PCOS patients must, in order to address their myriad symptoms. But like fatigue and sleeplessness, irritability could well have as its source not the PCOS itself but the drugs you may be using to combat its symptoms. It certainly also could be the hormonal imbalances that very commonly affect things like mood.

General irritability is not unlikely from the over-the-top concern you have with your health and the difficulty of controlling a multisymptom syndrome like PCOS. But if you feel your irritability is more deep than simply being frustrated with the condition, you will want to discuss it with your doctor and try to get to the source of the problem.

Mood swings and irritability can go hand in hand. Mood swings are associated directly with hormone imbalances; they're the classic symptom of women going through menopause, when the body's hormones are making significant adjustments to the slowing down and ending of the reproductive phase in a woman's life. Mood swings are also the territory of puberty—how many parents of preteen girls have you heard say, "She is so moody these days"? The imbalance of hormones characteristic of PCOS makes it logical that the syndrome would initiate moodiness and irritability in women who have it.

Until you gain real control of the hormonal issues your body is experiencing, you will need to use everything at your disposal to keep your moods from swinging to extremes. Learn to relax, call upon those favorite things that you do to relieve stress, make it a habit to count to ten before responding to an action or statement that a partner or family member does or says that might cause you to explode. Play with the dog or ride a horse, or do whatever you know helps to cheer you up when your moods take a downturn. It is not the cure for mood swings, but in the interim, while you create nutritional and chemical balances in your body, these are the kinds of things you have at your immediate disposal to help keep your moods in check.

Joint Pain

Some women with PCOS do complain of joint pain, but no specific correlation has been made. Certainly joint pain can be associated with lack of sleep and other issues that PCOS women face. If you are experiencing joint pain, you will want to work with your doctor to rule out arthritis, Lyme disease, or some other cause unrelated to PCOS.

Nausea

We've all heard of morning sickness during early pregnancy. Pregnancy causes a fluctuation in a woman's hormones, and morning sickness is the body's reaction to those fluctuations. Some women experience nausea during the monthly cycle. Again, this is due to the roller-coaster ride that the hormones are taking through a woman's body as her system works through the menstrual cycle. The same hormonal changes with PCOS can cause you to experience nausea.

Until your hormones get better balanced, you will need to address the symptom when it arises. You can help offset it by being careful what you eat during the times when you tend to become nauseous. To understand the timing, you will want to keep track of your bouts of nausea so you can be proactive about them.

As with other aspects of PCOS, make note of this in a journal. When the typical time frame is coming up for your nausea cycle to begin, try foods that can offset nausea, such as cinnamon, ginger, and peppermint.

Again, it can't be emphasized enough that the nausea you are experiencing may be unrelated to PCOS and should be monitored by and discussed with your doctor to rule out any other possible causes.

Depression

After reading the last chapter on the primary symptoms and this chapter on the secondary symptoms, it is pretty easy to see why the woman with PCOS might become depressed. This is a lot of complicated and often contradictory symptoms to deal with! It can be simply overwhelming to spend so much effort and time tackling the many symptoms that can be thrown at the PCOS patient all at once. And if you are dealing with extreme weight problems, you can't even turn to comfort foods to help cheer you up, because even though you eat almost nothing, you still can't shed a pound. This can almost seem like too much to bear.

Don't ignore depression, whatever you think the cause. Be sure to tell your doctor if you feel you are significantly down. Before deciding that the daunting task of sorting out all of these health issues is the cause of your depression, you and your doctor will want to check out other possibilities, to determine that something more specific isn't causing it.

Of course, hormones out of balance will be a big factor. Menopause and premenstrual syndrome are conditions that are commonly known to send women into a funk with depression-like symptoms. But there are many other things that can cause depression as well.

If you are taking medications, whether they are related to tackling PCOS or not, talk them over with your doctor. Some drugs can cause mild depression. You may have to do some trial and error to experiment and find the cause, but don't just stop taking a prescribed drug to find out if it is making you depressed; discuss with your doctor the possibility of stopping the drug, perhaps temporarily. There are several drugs that you must wean yourself from in stages, not just stop cold turkey.

Depression may not be a common side effect of a particular drug, but perhaps that is what it does to you; you may even be allergic to the medication or one of its ingredients. Everyone is different. Don't decide that a drug is not the culprit just because depression isn't written on the bottle as a possible side effect.

Finding the cause of your depression may take some time—even if something specific, such as a drug, doesn't come up as a cause—but it's important to keep trying. See a counselor, therapist, family counselor, or psychologist, and begin to work through your depression. It may be due to something in your life in general, not health-related at all, that is bringing you down. You will need all the physical and mental energy you can muster to get control of PCOS, so it is important to deal with depression.

Sometimes when women are dealing with PCOS they are so focused on this particular complicated condition that they forget that something else could be going on in their bodies. With PCOS having so many facets, it's frustrating to think that you will need to deal with an unrelated health issue, but the rest of your body is subject to many problems as well. You will need to work a little extra hard to keep up with your overall health outside the bounds of PCOS.

Life can be good despite a diagnosis of PCOS!

A PERSONAL STORY

Bridget

PCOS began to surface in Bridget's life in the classic way with the classic symptoms: never establishing a regular menstrual cycle from the time she started her period at twelve and a constant battle with weight control. Both of the problems, she and her family and her doctors felt, were easily traced to their source.

The irregular menstrual cycle one was simple: Girls take a while to establish their cycles. In other words, the prevailing wisdom is that it's normal for a girl in her teens to have "abnormal" periods.

The obesity piece was perhaps not as simple, but everyone felt it was explainable: Her mom and dad were both "larger sized," and Bridget was one of six children. "We didn't have the money to eat well, to eat fancy foods," Bridget remembers.

The one symptom that was not easily explained was the excessive hair growth. Embarrassed by her weight and dark facial hair, and teased about it by other kids, Bridget dealt with the situation by simply staying at home. There was no lack of things to do there—her father worked two jobs, her mother worked a forty-hour week as a nurse, and she was the second oldest of six kids. There was laundry, housework, and various other chores that build up fast in a big household. And when she wasn't taking care of those things, she locked herself in her room and wrote poetry. This sedentary part of her lifestyle, combined with a carbohydrate-heavy diet, was the cause of her obesity, according to her doctors.

At age fourteen, Bridget saw her doctor about her symptoms. The doctor sent her to an endocrinologist, looking for conditions such as Cushing's disease and other hormonal problems. Bridget was given renal exams and had lots of blood work done. Ultimately, the doctor put her on Provera (a hormone treatment that corrects for progesterone deficiency) between ages fifteen and sixteen. It didn't help anything, and so she was taken off it. With renal tests coming out normal and a normal thyroid, she was put on birth control to regulate her periods, but her high blood pressure couldn't take it.

When she graduated from high school in 1985, at age seventeen, Bridget saw some improvement. She moved out of her parents' home and lived on her own. With little money and no car, she walked everywhere. She got a lot of exercise, ate minimal amounts, and lost eighty pounds!

But the weight loss did not seem to have much of a positive effect on her PCOS symptoms. Her periods were still irregular, and now her doctor was saying it was because she was getting too much exercise. How could she win?

In 1991, with her weight still at a low level, she experienced terrific pain in her lower-right abdomen area. She was working for an OB/GYN, who diagnosed it as an ovarian torsion, for which Bridget underwent surgery to straighten the ovary. The reason the twisted ovary could not straighten itself? There were so many exterior cysts from PCOS, it basically got stuck.

Throughout all of this, Bridget's insulin level was fine. When she visited a naturopathic doctor, he was certain they would find high insulin levels. When the test that he did in the office came out with insulin at perfect levels, he thought it was a fluke. He waited a while and did the test again, with almost the exact same results.

With all of her classic symptoms, her long-term relationship with PCOS, and her determination to change her symptoms, it would be a safe assumption that Bridget would be totally focused on solving the PCOS problem. However, life has a way of keeping us on our toes, and Bridget has been dealt a number of health issues that have put PCOS pretty far into the background.

Bridget now works as an office manager in a busy holistic health practice. She enjoys her job and makes a good living that enables her to live a good life.

"Now that I make decent money," she laughs, "I treat myself to nice dinners and my weight is still a problem."

Bridget hasn't had a period in five years and is concerned she will never have kids. She's not even sure she wants to have children, but she'd at least like to be able to consider it. Although she is not currently in a relationship, her doctor has told her that now is the time to start dealing with her fertility issues. It will take a while to get on track, so she needs to start now to make changes and be ready when she is ready to consider children.

CHAPTER FIVE ∽

Medical Treatment for PCOS
Drugs and Surgical Options

There are a number of medications that can be effective for the treatment of PCOS symptoms and the prevention of long-term complications. The key is that the choice of medications must be individualized, according to the treatment goals for a given individual. For some women, the most bothersome concern is unwanted facial hair growth, while for others the primary issue is infertility, and for yet others weight gain is most annoying, frustrating, and hard to get under control.

Each of these symptoms can be treated with a different set of medications. If there is evidence of underlying insulin resistance, despite appropriate lifestyle interventions and self-help measures, then medications used for the treatment of type 2 diabetes can be beneficial for both treatment of symptoms and prevention of long-term complications.

It would take a complete book to list all of the medical treatments, but the following sections list the main options that we will discuss in association with specific treatment goals for PCOS:

Antiandrogen Medications
• Testosterone receptor blockers
    • Aldactone (spironolactone)
    • Cyproterone acetate (not available in the U.S.)
    • Tagamet (cimetidine)

Androgens are male hormones such as testosterone and its derivatives. Medicines in this category are structurally similar to testosterone but possess no testosterone-like properties. Because of this similarity, they can attach themselves to testosterone receptors in the cells and thus prevent the receptors from being stimulated by testosterone. Although testosterone can inhibit growth of hair follicles in the scalp, it stimulates facial/body hair growth and increases production of sebum in the oily sebaceous glands of the skin. So antiandrogen medications are used to treat symptoms related to acne, male-pattern baldness, and facial hair growth and other male-type hair growth on the body.

• Testosterone metabolism blockers
    • Propecia (finasteride)
    • Dutasteride (soon to be released)

These medicines prevent conversion of the less active testosterone to a stronger form called dihydrotestosterone (DHT). Initially prescribed to treat enlargement of the prostate, they have been found to decrease male-pattern hair loss. The product information states that women should not use Propecia and that they shouldn't even touch crushed or damaged tablets if they are of child-bearing age. Despite these warnings, Propecia has been used successfully by women with male-pattern hair loss.

• Eulexin (flutamide)

This is one of the strongest antiandrogen medicines available and consequently also has the most potential for serious side effects (such as liver damage). The precise mechanism of action of the antitestosterone effect of flutamide is not well understood. The FDA-approved use of this drug is for men with prostate cancer, and labeling states that it is not for use in women. Prescribing of flutamide for women with PCOS, despite the lack of FDA approval, is an example of an "off-label" use. Topical solutions of flutamide appear to hold promise for scalp hair loss with less risk of side effects.

All of the antiandrogen medications used for women with PCOS are prescribed in an off-label fashion. This does not mean these medicines are ineffective, but it does mean that the pharmaceutical companies have not done the extensive research on safety and efficacy needed to receive FDA approval for treatment of PCOS-related symptoms with these drugs. None of these medications should be used during pregnancy or by nursing women, as they can alter development of the fetus or newborn. Because of the irregular and unpredictable menstrual cycles associated with PCOS, these medicines should be used with contraceptives in women who are sexually active. Because contraceptives are not 100 percent reliable, some would argue that the potential risks of antiandrogens can only be justified in women who have had a tuboligation (tubes tied) or a hysterectomy.

Antidiabetic Medications
• "Insulin-sparing" agents (theoretic, but as yet undocumented, benefit)
• "Starch blockers"
    • Precose (acarbose)
    • Glyset (miglitol)

These medicines are taken with the first bite of each meal. By inhibiting an enzyme (alpha-glucosidase) needed to digest carbohydrates, they cause a decrease in absorption of sugar into the bloodstream from the intestinal tract. Less incoming sugar means that your body needs to produce less insulin. Since increased insulin production worsens the hormonal imbalances of PCOS, taking medicines that decrease insulin requirements should (in theory) be helpful, though research to confirm this has not yet been done. The most common side effects of these medicines (or any medicines that impair normal digestion and absorption of foods) are gas or diarrhea. Starting at the lowest possible dose of medicine generally minimizes these side effects, and the dose can be gradually increased as tolerated.

- "Insulin sensitizers" (documented benefit)
- Biguanides
    - Glucophage (metformin)
- Thiazolidinediones
    - Actos (pioglitazone)
    - Avandia (rosiglitazone)

Insulin sensitizers allow the available insulin in your body to work more effectively. Based on head-to-head comparisons of these two classes of insulin sensitizers, metformin appears to be most useful. Combining metformin with one of the thiazolidinediones does not appear to confer any additional significant therapeutic benefits. One of the advantages of metformin is that it is often associated with weight loss, while the thiazolidinediones are usually associated with weight gain.

- "Insulin boosters" (counterproductive)
    - Sulfonylureas
    - Meglitinides

You might think that all antidiabetic medications should be helpful for patients with PCOS if insulin resistance is the underlying problem. However, since the hormonal imbalances of PCOS are exacerbated by the body's compensatory increase in insulin production, taking medications that further increase pancreatic insulin production would only make things worse and risk causing hypoglycemia (dangerously low blood sugar). The only appropriate application of insulin boosters for women with PCOS would be for those who have progressed to frank diabetes, in which the body's compensatory mechanisms are not enough to control blood sugar. Even in this decompensated situation, insulin boosters would be a last choice, and should be tried only if diet, exercise, insulin-sparing agents, and insulin-sensitizers have proven inadequate.

None of the antidiabetic medicines have been FDA-approved yet for use in patients with PCOS. The longstanding tradition of prescribing off-label uses for medicines is widespread, and in many cases there are more unofficial uses than officially recognized and endorsed indications.

Gonadotropin-Releasing Hormone Antagonists
• Lupron (leuprolide)

This synthetic imitation of gonadotropin-releasing hormone (produced by the hypothalamus to stimulate LH and FSH production by the pituitary gland) causes an initial transient rise in FSH, then a precipitous decline of both FSH and LH when the pituitary gland stops responding to the fake hormone. Since chronically elevated LH levels prevent ovulation and stimulate production of testosterone by the ovaries, the use of Lupron can help restore more normal ovarian function. Lupron is often used as part of an infertility treatment program, to prepare the ovaries for a better response to the ovulation-inducing medicines. Currently the only FDA-approved uses for Lupron are to treat men with prostate cancer and women with endometriosis or uterine fibroids. Therefore, the use of Lupron for infertility in women (with or without PCOS) is yet another example of an off-label use.

Hair-Growth Stimulators
• Rogaine solution (minoxidil)

Minoxidil tablets were developed to treat patients with elevated blood pressure. Minoxidil lowers blood pressure by dilating blood vessels. A side effect noted in patients with high blood pressure is that many had increased hair growth. In order to help hair growth without bottoming out blood pressure in patients with normal blood pressure, a weak (2 percent) topical formulation was developed. Initially this was available only by prescription, but Rogaine is now available as an over-the-counter product. Rogaine has been used successfully by both men and women to treat hair loss. This medication has to be applied twice daily for at least four to eight months to see results, and any benefits are lost after discontinuation.

Hair Metabolism Inhibitors
• Vaniqa cream (eflornithine)

Vaniqa dramatically slows unwanted facial hair growth by inhibiting an enzyme (ornithine decarboxylase) that is important for metabolism of the cells in hair follicles. Since Vaniqa doesn't remove unwanted hairs but simply slows down their growth, some method of hair removal (electrolysis, plucking, shaving) also needs to be used (though much less frequently than would otherwise be necessary).

Menstrual Regulators
• Progestins
• Synthetic
     • Amen/Cycrin/Provera (medroxyprogesterone)

- Bioidentical
    - Prometrium (progesterone)

Synthetic progestins (progesterone-like compounds) have been prescribed and studied more extensively than natural progesterone. However, based on available research, progesterone appears to provide all the same benefits with fewer side effects than medroxyprogesterone. When women with PCOS neither ovulate nor subsequently develop a corpus luteum, they become progesterone-deficient. This progesterone deficiency allows the endometrial lining of the uterus to become abnormally thick under the unopposed influence of estrogen. The normal cyclic rise and fall of progesterone responsible for healthy shedding of the endometrium, and associated menstrual flow, can be mimicked with the use of cyclic progestins.

- Birth-control pills

Birth-control pills inhibit ovulation but also provide cyclic progestin stimulation to simulate a normal and predictable menstrual cycle. There are a variety of different birth-control pills that use different estrogen derivatives and progestins. There is even a weekly contraceptive patch now available, but its use specifically in women with PCOS has not been studied yet. It makes sense to choose contraceptives with progestins that are the least androgenic (such as desogestrel or norgestimate) to regulate the menstrual cycle.

Ovulation Inducers
- Clomid/Serophene (clomiphene)
- Pergonal/Humegon/Repronex (hMG)
- Follistim/Gonal F (FSH)
- Profasi/Pregnyl (HCG)

While these agents can be very helpful to induce ovulation in women with infertility caused by PCOS, it is common for multiple eggs to be released. The challenges and complications of multiple pregnancies in this case would need to be handled by an obstetrician and a perinatologist/neonatologist specializing in high-risk pregnancies.

Surgery
• Ovarian wedge resection
• Laparoscopic ovarian drilling

Although surgical procedures are used far less frequently now that a number of effective medicines are available, there are still times when surgery can be useful. Reducing the tissue mass (wedge resection) of an abnormal polycystic ovary that is producing high amounts of testosterone can improve symptoms of androgen excess and also increase the chances of ovulation. Laparoscopic ovarian drilling sounds like a terrible industrial procedure, but it is actually less invasive than the older technique of wedge resection. When the two procedures are compared, laparoscopic ovarian drilling seems to provide superior outcomes.

Treatment Goals
Acne/Unwanted Hair Growth/Hair Loss
Weight loss can improve insulin resistance and decrease levels of androgens, thereby indirectly improving acne, unwanted facial/body hair (hirsutism), and male-pattern hair loss (alopecia androgenetica). Aside from appropriate dietary measures and exercise, the use of prescription weight-loss aids (such as phentermine, Meridia/sibutramine, or Xenical/orlistat) may be beneficial in some situations. Prescribing a weight-loss medication to treat acne, hirsutism, or alopecia may at first glance seem counterintuitive or perhaps even inappropriate. However, an understanding of the underlying physiology responsible

for the symptoms makes it clear that this can indeed be an effective and appropriate treatment strategy for women with PCOS, obesity, and insulin resistance.

A much more obvious and direct approach to treating acne and un-wanted hair would involve the use of "anti-acne" and "anti-hair" medications. Examples of anti-acne medications include topical cleansers to decrease oiliness, keratolytics (such as benzoyl peroxide or azelaic acid) to clear out pores, astringents to tighten pores, topi-cal or oral antibiotics to decrease skin bacteria, and topical or oral agents that alter the growth and/or shedding of skin cells (such as Retin-A/Avita/tretinoin, Tazorac/tazarotene, Differin/adapalene, or Accutane/isotretinoin). Vaniqa cream (eflornithine), an inhibitor of hair growth, is the only example we currently have of an anti-hair medicine. While using dermatologic (skin) interventions may be some-what useful, the acne or hirsutism in this situation is not primarily a skin problem. The acne and hirsutism of PCOS are really superficial manifestations of excessive male hormones.

It is eminently logical to use antiandrogen medications to treat acne, hirsutism, and alopecia associated with elevated androgens. These medications do reduce symptoms of androgen excess, but they en-hance infertility and are generally not helpful to correct menstrual irregularities, reduce the risk of endometrial cancer associated with PCOS, or decrease insulin resistance. Therefore, the antiandrogen medications can be considered fairly unidimensional in their useful-ness. The antiandrogens are contraindicated during pregnancy, and women of childbearing age must use contraception with these medi-cines if sexually active.

Another option available for male-pattern hair loss is the use of topical Rogaine to stimulate scalp hair growth. The response rates commonly quoted for Rogaine are that about 50-60 percent of users will have a positive response, with a third of these having good hair growth, a third having moderate hair growth, and a third having minimal (classic "peach fuzz") growth. Even the one in five to one in six who do have a good response can expect to lose the gains made if they stop using Rogaine.

Weight Gain/Insulin Resistance

Dietary measures and exercise, as discussed in the treatment of acne, hirsutism, and alopecia, are obviously a first step to facilitate weight loss and decrease insulin resistance (less sugar going from the bloodstream into the cells in response to insulin secreted by the pancreas). Similarly, it doesn't take much creativity to see how prescription weight-loss medications might play a positive role, if diet and exercise alone are not achieving adequate results. The use of antidiabetic medications in patients with PCOS who do not meet the diagnostic criteria for diabetes requires a little more imagination.

Patients with PCOS, whether overweight or not, initially have normal blood-sugar readings despite their insulin resistance. These normal blood sugars are achieved by a metabolic sleight of hand in which the body compensates for insulin resistance by producing more insulin. The ability of the body to maintain this hyperinsulinemic state decreases over time as the overworked pancreas struggles to keep up with increasing insulin demands. When the pancreas can no longer keep up, decompensation occurs and the blood sugars finally begin to rise to the point where there is an abnormal glucose tolerance test. Eventually, if this course of events continues unabated, the sugar readings become elevated enough to qualify for an official diagnosis of type 2 diabetes. Once a patient has been diagnosed with diabetes, everyone and their dog (assuming the dog went to medical school) is ready to prescribe antidiabetic medications—but prescribing antidiabetic medications to

PCOS patients with normal blood sugars involves a more subtle thought process.

Since insulin resistance and compensatory hyperinsulinemia are thought to be the underlying cause of PCOS in many instances, the use of some of the newer antidiabetic medications (insulin sensitizers and insulin-sparing agents) can have dramatic and far-reaching effects. For instance, the use of Glucophage/metformin in patients with PCOS has been shown to decrease androgen levels, improve acne and hirsutism, normalize irregular menstrual cycles, restore fertility, facilitate weight loss, and prevent progression to diabetes. The appropriate use of antidiabetic medications not only treats virtually all of the symptoms of PCOS, it also prevents the most serious complication. Conversely, the inappropriate use of older antidiabetic medications (insulin boosters) would be expected to worsen the symptoms of PCOS and accelerate the development of complications.

Irregular Menstrual Cycles

Depending on the woman, the decreased frequency of menstrual cycles and the irregular bleeding associated with PCOS can be a significant nuisance or a minor inconvenience. Regardless of the perceived level of inconvenience, the irregular menstrual cycles are linked to an increased risk of endometrial cancer. The normal cyclic shedding of the endometrium (inner lining of the uterus), which ensues from the rise and fall of progesterone production by the corpus luteum following ovulation, is impaired in women with PCOS. The result is that the endometrium can become abnormally thickened due to unopposed stimulation by estrogen for long periods of time. These conditions increase the risk of endometrial cancer and underscore the need for preventive screening through regular gynecologic checkups in women with PCOS. With this understanding, it becomes apparent that treating irregular menstrual cycles is more than a matter of convenience. Inducing regular, cyclic shedding of the uterine lining in women with PCOS will actually lower their risk of developing endometrial cancer.

The most commonly used strategy to induce a regular menstrual cycle is to prescribe birth-control pills. There are over forty pills to choose from, each with a slightly different blend of estrogens and progestins. Since it makes sense to use progestins with the least androgenic activity (desogestrel or norgestimate), this narrows the field to a more manageable eight choices: Apri, Desogen, Kariva, Mircette, Ortho-Cept, Ortho-Cyclen, Ortho Tri-Cyclen, or Ortho Tri-Cyclen Lo.

Another option that has been used to induce cyclic shedding of the endometrium is prescribing progestins for ten to fourteen days out of each month. Since cyclic use of progestins does not prevent ovulation, it cannot be used as a contraceptive. Use of progestins during pregnancy is contraindicated (with rare exceptions), and therefore measures to avoid pregnancy must be used in women using cyclic progestins. Although synthetic medoxyprogesterone (Amen/Cycrin/Provera) has historically been the most commonly prescribed progestin, there is increasing evidence that using bioidentical (synthetic compounds chemically indistinguishable from compounds produced by the human body) progesterone (available through compounding pharmacies and also as "Prometrium") may be preferable.

Infertility

The treatment of infertility is complex and multifactorial. Effective treatment of infertility, perhaps as much as any field of medicine, is both an art and a science and must address the subtle and intangible qualities of humanity as well as precise parameters of biochemistry. Infertility specialists can have dramatically different success rates based on their experience and the specific protocols and treatments they use.

Therefore one of the most important choices in handling infertility is the decision of which doctor to work with.

Infertility in women with PCOS is classically due to lack of ovulation or infrequent/irregular ovulation. If this is the case, the use of gonadotropin-releasing hormone antagonists (such as Lupron/leuprolide) followed by ovulation-inducing agents (such as clomiphene, hMG, FSH, or HCG) can facilitate conception. The possibility of multiple conceptions/multiple pregnancies with these regimens requires close monitoring and expert management. In women with PCOS who have not responded to these complex regimens, the use of an insulin sensitizer (such as Glucophage/metformin) has been shown to improve outcomes.

The obvious question that arises then (since hyperinsulinemia may be the underlying cause of the hormonal imbalances and lack of ovulation) is: Why not start by first addressing the hyperinsulinemia, rather than turning to this as a last resort? Diet, exercise, weight loss (if overweight), and insulin-sparing/sensitizing agents (if needed) are indeed a logical place to begin, if hyperinsulinemia is the main culprit responsible for infertility. If this approach is inadequate, then moving on to the gonadotropic-releasing hormone antagonists and ovulation inducers may be appropriate. If all else fails, then surgical interventions such as an ovarian wedge resection or laparoscopic ovarian drilling may achieve the desired results. These surgical techniques may, in fact, be beneficial for any of the symptoms associated with PCOS. However, since the risk/benefit ratio of lifestyle interventions and/or medications is generally more favorable, these surgical interventions are usually a last choice.

A Few Words About Insurance

The treatment of infertility is not covered by many health insurance companies. Similarly, many insurance companies will exclude covering medicines prescribed for "off-label" uses. As described in this chapter, many effective treatments for acne/hirsutism/alopecia/ weight gain/irregular menses/infertility in women with PCOS are off-label uses of medicines that are FDA-approved for other conditions. While medical knowledge has advanced significantly in regard to the treatment of patients with PCOS, insurance reimbursement is not yet equally enlightened. Not paying for weight-loss medicines and insulin sensitizers in a woman with PCOS whose primary complaint is acne may save the insurance company money in the short run, but it will end up costing the insurance company and the patient a lot more in the long run, when complications of diabetes develop down the road. Therefore, even if efforts to get the insurance company to pay are not fruitful, I would encourage you to pay out of pocket (if at all possible) to do what it takes to prevent the development of diabetes.

A recurrent theme of this book is that the symptoms of PCOS provide an early warning of hyperinsulinemia and an ideal opportunity to prevent serious medical problems. Refusing to prescribe (or buy and use) a medicine (or a gym membership and weight-loss program) that can prevent diabetes because it's not covered by health insurance is short-sighted. In order to capitalize on the opportunity for prevention that PCOS offers, doctors and their patients may at times need to be more enlightened than insurance company executives.

A PERSONAL STORY

Tracy

At around age twelve, Tracy developed a dark patch of skin on her inner thigh. She thought it must be a birthmark, although she had never noticed it before. This secondary symptom of PCOS, called *acanthosis nigricans,* was Tracy's first real red flag of the syndrome—she just didn't know it yet.

She had started her menstrual cycle at the very young age of nine, but her cycles were irregular right from the beginning. By age sixteen she had extreme difficulties, including bleeding lasting for weeks instead of the usual days. Her doctor did a laparoscopic exam and found "thousands" of little cysts on her ovaries. PCOS was the diagnosis.

The doctor recommended that Tracy take birth-control pills to regulate her cycle, which she did for five years, from age sixteen to age twenty-one. Her periods did regulate for a while. Then at age eighteen she first began to notice an increased amount of facial hair.

Tracy married, and by age twenty-two wanted to start a family. She could not get pregnant. Her doctor did blood work and examined her reproductive anatomy for problems—and declared Tracy to be just fine.

Finally, at age twenty-six, Tracy tried the drug Clomid (whose scientific name is clomiphene citrate), a fertility drug used to induce ovulation. She did just one cycle of Clomid and decided that if she was going to get pregnant, she was, and if not, she wasn't.

At age thirty-eight, Tracy was still not pregnant, and weighed 185 pounds at a five-foot height. Tracy had already found that in order to lose any weight at all, she needed to quite literally starve herself; she tried that once and lost sixty-five pounds, but the minute she started eating again, she quickly gained it back. She decided she had absolutely no intention of starving herself or developing eating disorders, so she simply tried to eat as healthfully as she could and stopped worrying about her weight.

Tracy had heard lots of success stories about women who used metformin, so she insisted to her doctor that she try it. One day, eight months into her metformin regimen, a pregnancy test came out positive. Tracy was stunned.

She ran to the pharmacy and asked the pharmacist if metformin could give her a false positive reading. The pharmacist told her that the EPT tests are 99 percent accurate. Tracy went to another pharmacy and asked the pharmacist the same question. When she got the same answer, she bought another test and went home.

She tried the second test. Another positive.

Tracy, at the time of this interview, was four and a half months pregnant and ecstatic. She stopped the metformin as suggested, twelve weeks into her pregnancy. She continues to watch what she eats, although she admits she isn't as dedicated about exercising as she feels she should be.

"PCOS has been hard to deal with from a social standpoint," she admits. "The self-esteem issues are so hard. I couldn't understand why God would give me a pretty face but put facial hair on it. But the only thing I have ever really wanted was to have a child." And that is where all of Tracy's focus is now.

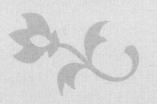

CHAPTER SIX ∿

The First Step for Success in Managing PCOS
Diet, Nutrition, and Weight Control

Have you been told by your doctor that you need to lose weight? Or need to lose *more* weight? And did you feel like responding, "No kidding!"? Most people who are overweight don't need to be told they need to lose weight. However, perhaps even more frustrating is that you want to say, "But I don't eat anything now; how can I eat less?" This is one of the key exasperating dilemmas facing PCOS patients.

Weight control for women with PCOS can be a major turning point for keeping other symptoms at bay. But the very symptoms that can be alleviated by weight control, and the ways that some symptoms are best alleviated, can be contributing factors to weight gain in the first place.

Some women develop eating disorders such as anorexia and bulimia in a desperate attempt to get their weight under control. If you have despaired over weight issues and find that you are going down the eating disorder road, please get medical help immediately. The purging and starving that are the hallmarks of these disorders are not healthy solutions to weight problems, and they can lead to life-threatening health issues. While the weight loss caused by eating disorders can seem as if it is helping your weight problems, the havoc they wreak on your body's overall health and well-being actually will eventually cause other PCOS symptoms to worsen—and cause you to have other health problems to deal with, which is the last thing you need.

Causes for Weight Gain in PCOS Patients: The Hormone Connection

The theme you may notice repeating throughout this book is that once you start to gain control of the underlying problems of your PCOS, the symptoms will subside, including your excess weight.

A lot of these underlying problems usually relate to hormones. An out-of-balance endocrine system throws off the way your body utilizes nourishment, and therefore the food you eat is not processed in the most efficient manner. Carbohydrates, for instance, are a great source of immediate energy to most people, but in your body they may be turned directly into stored energy, in the form of fat. When insulin resistance causes your body's hormones to react the opposite to what is desirable—that is, you store energy as fat rather than burn it off—you are going to have weight problems and inevitably get caught between the proverbial rock and a hard place. This is where the specifics of your diet kick in.

High levels of insulin in your body trigger other hormonal responses, such as an increase in androgens, and more specifically testosterone. This alone can cause irregular cycles, since the excess testosterone sends messages to the ovaries not to release an egg, and—voila!—you have no period. Many of the other frustrating symptoms experienced by women with PCOS, such as baldness, excess hair growth, and acne, are also androgen-related. What is the logical way to counteract this? Make sure your body is not set up to stimulate the androgens in the first place. The best way to do that? Be precise about your diet.

The Apple and the Pear

Weight gain in women is often described as creating an apple-shaped or a pear-shaped outline. In a pear-shaped body, the weight gain is around the buttocks and thighs. In an apple-shaped body, the weight gain is concentrated around the middle of the body. Studies have shown this apple shape to be the more prone to significant health issues such as heart disease, high blood pressure, diabetes, and certain cancers. PCOS women who are overweight tend to be of the apple-shaped weight-gain type, making it yet another reason to be diet-conscious and begin a weight-loss plan.

You probably didn't expect to be a professional juggler, but once you have been diagnosed with PCOS, you begin to realize how many balls you need to have in the air in order to stay ahead of all the various symptoms related to this disorder!

Become a Nutrition Expert

Despite the success or lack of success of any dieting programs you have tried, and despite the fact that many other things need to balance out in order for any of your weight-loss attempts to have an impact, it is important to be working on a good diet. Perhaps you have reduced your calorie intake and been on the mark with portion control, but if what you are eating isn't the best nutrition for the functioning of your body, you can manage calories and portions all you want and see no weight-loss results.

This isn't to say that what you are eating is bad; it just may not constitute the best nutrition for your chemical makeup, given the PCOS factor. When your other diet- and weight-related symptoms begin to work themselves out, you want to be poised to lose weight, not to have to catch up to good eating at that point.

You don't want to finally find the right treatment to balance your hormones and then start to practice excellent eating habits. If you start practicing good eating and balanced nutrition right now, you will see quick results in the weight-loss department when the things that have been fighting against you are under control.

You don't have to become so fanatical about nutrition that you get a chemistry set and analyze the chemical makeup of every item of food before you put it in your mouth. But you do want to understand the principles of good nutrition as well as the reasons behind phenomena like the proverbial "sweet tooth" and salt addictions.

Once you begin to be more conscious of nutrition and the effects that certain foods have on your body, it becomes a bit of an addiction in itself. And once you change your eating habits, your body's metabolism starts to change, and you won't even be tempted by things that won't help your weight-control program. To top it all off, once you begin to lose a few pounds, that in itself will become motivation to stick to your regimen.

The Basics of Good Nutrition

While you probably won't run out and get a degree in dietary science, there are some basics that all adults should know about the food we eat, how our bodies utilize that food, and what our bodies need in order to function optimally. And when you are faced with a health concern like PCOS, you will want to learn a little more than the average adult about nutrition. Many diseases and disorders—diabetes perhaps the most commonly known one—are greatly affected by a person's eating habits and food choices.

In the United States, the American Dietetic Association (and in Canada, the ADA's counterpart, the CDA) is a major source of dietary information and guidelines. Although there are forty nutrients that food provides us, they are divided into the following six groups (plus water):

> *Carbohydrates:* Your body gets its energy from carbohydrates. Simple carbohydrates are obtained in the form of sugars providing immediate energy, while complex carbohydrates come into the body in the form of starch and are processed by the digestive system into usable energy by the body. Simple carbohydrates tend to be digested and absorbed more quickly than the same amount of calories from complex carbohydrates. This means that simple carbohydrates will make your blood sugar spike faster and higher than the same amount of calories from complex carbohydrates. The "glycemic index" of a food is a reflection of how much that food raises your blood sugar. Simple carbohydrates usually have a higher glycemic index than complex carbohydrates. High glycemic-index foods demand a more vigorous insulin response from your pancreas. Therefore, if you are already having problems with insulin resistance associated with your PCOS, a high glycemic-index diet will tend to make your condition worse. In light of this, choosing to follow a low glycemic-index diet can be particularly useful for patients with PCOS.
>
> However, there is more to the glycemic index than many things you read would lead you to believe. The tendency is to say that all high glycemic foods are bad for you, are the cause of the impending downfall of Western society, and should be avoided.

Carrots have a high glycemic index—should you eliminate carrots from your diet? Absolutely not! Carrots provide many important nutrients and are part of a healthy diet. Because carrots have a very low "calorie density," you would have to eat huge quantities of them to have much impact on your blood-sugar and insulin responses. Conversely, eating lots of cheese, which has a low glycemic index but a high calorie density, can contribute to weight gain that in turn leads to worsening of insulin resistance.

Carrots and cheese are good examples of the folly of fixating on the glycemic index to the exclusion of other important factors. For weight loss and decreased demands for insulin from your pancreas, the best strategy is to eat mostly foods that are both low in calories and low on their glycemic index. The other thing to consider is that eating thirty pounds per day of food is not going to work, even if it is the healthiest, lowest-calorie, lowest glycemic-index food in the world. The key is moderation in all things, and letting an awareness of the glycemic index of foods influence your food choices without imposing needlessly rigid and arbitrary constraints.

Fiber: Fiber is not digested or absorbed but plays a crucial role in nutrition. Fiber is generally categorized as soluble or insoluble, with proven health benefits from both types. Fiber is known to decrease the absorption of fats and slow the absorption of sugars. Because of the delaying effect on absorption, fiber lowers the glycemic index of any carbohydrates consumed. In addition to keeping your bowels regular, lowering your cholesterol, and helping you feel full (so you're less likely to overeat), fiber tends to reduce your insulin requirements. Fiber is your friend. Good sources of fiber include most fruits and vegetables, beans, peas, and whole grains. Throwing your fruits and/or vegetables into the blender/juicer decreases some of the inherent benefits of fiber and instantly raises the glycemic index of the food by allowing you to process and absorb it more quickly. Even though fiber is your friend, the friendship is not always harmonious. Some people are particularly sensitive and experience uncomfortable bloating and intestinal gas when they dramatically increase their fiber intake. The notorious gas-producing properties of beans can be minimized by soaking them overnight, discarding the excess water, rinsing, and then boiling. A product like beano® that contains the enzyme alpha-galactosidase can cut gas production for some people. Gradually increasing your fiber intake over several weeks to months is another way to reduce gas problems. If you choose to use a fiber supplement in addition to consuming more high-fiber foods, be sure to take any medicines an hour before or two hours after the fiber supplement, to ensure that the medicine will be well absorbed.

Fats: With the proliferation of discussions about cholesterol, you'd almost have to live in a cave to avoid having heard of saturated and unsaturated fats. First, cholesterol is required by your body to perform many functions important to hormones and nutrient use. However, the human body makes all the cholesterol it needs; any extra cholesterol in the body is converted to fat. Saturated fats also contain dietary cholesterol. Excess cholesterol in the bloodstream can collect around the walls of the arteries, causing arteriosclerosis and increasing the risk of a heart attack or stroke. Apart from decreasing intake of saturated fats (from animal sources and hydrogenated oils in processed foods), another wise move is to make sure that the fats you do consume are predominantly health-promoting unsaturated fats such as olive oil (monounsaturated) and flax or cold-water fish oils (omega-3 polyunsaturated). Fats are the most concentrated source of calories (twice as many calories per gram as either carbohydrates or proteins) and should be consumed sparingly. A little bit of fat can go a long way to enhance the taste and texture of meals. Another, often unrecognized, benefit of fats is that they tend to slow the rate of digestion and absorption of your food, thereby lowering the glycemic index and decreasing the roller-coaster demand for insulin. So while being conscious of the calories, it is both possible and desirable to consume small amounts of healthy fats, even as you are adhering to a dietary regimen that promotes weight loss.

Proteins: Amino acids build and repair body tissue and are critical to good health. Proteins supply amino acids to our bodies. Proteins also supply an energy boost if the body doesn't have other energy supplies to draw on.

Vitamins: Each vitamin has a different critical function in the body. They are responsible for the chemical reactions that take place, making our bodies work the way they are supposed to. Multivitamins are a good thing to take if you feel your diet is lacking; however, the best way to bring vitamins into our bodies is via the foods we eat.

Minerals: Minerals, like vitamins, have several key roles in the proper functioning of the human body. Perhaps the best known of the minerals is calcium, well known for its role in bone development and health. Many other minerals are required only in trace amounts, but are still critical to human health.

Water: Water is also essential to nutrition. Although some have questioned the benefits of the old rule of thumb that we should drink eight 8-ounce glasses of water each day, there remains no question that water is a key requirement for health. Recently published research has documented that men who drink five or more 8-ounce glasses of water daily have significantly fewer heart attacks than those who drink two or fewer glasses of water per day. Although this same research has not yet been done with women, there is no reason to suspect that the results would be any different. The mechanism for this benefit of water consumption appears to be that dehydration increases the tendency for blood to clot and, conversely, that adequate hydration prevents excessive blood clotting. Blood clotting is a risk factor for heart disease that is decreased by sufficient water intake. Viewed in this light, adequate water intake can actually be a matter of life and death! Body weight is over half and as much as 75 percent water. Water regulates your body temperature, it helps the nutrients you take in to reach their destinations, and it helps clear byproducts in the form of waste out of your system. You can decide for yourself how much to drink in a day, but just don't forget about the importance of water!

Without even understanding the specifics of the essential nutrients your body needs to function properly, you can be confident you are getting these nutrients by being sure to follow these dietary guidelines for daily servings from the United States Department of Agriculture:

- 2-3 servings of meat, fish, eggs, beans, or nuts (1 egg, ½ cup beans, or a meat/fish portion the size of a deck of cards).
- 2-3 servings of milk, yogurt, or cheese (2 ounces cheese or 1 cup milk/yogurt). You can substitute nondairy products like soy milk if you cannot eat dairy.
- 4-6 servings of whole grains (1 slice bread, ½ cup rice/pasta, 1 bowl cereal).
- 4 fruit servings (1 piece of fruit equals one serving).
- 5 vegetable servings (½ cup each).
- Moderate amounts of oils and fats.

Avoid sugared cereals, canned fruit in heavy syrup, salted chips, and other prepared foods that sneak in excess salt or sugar that you don't need.

Using a Registered Dietitian

You can start right off simply by changing the eating habits that you know are working against you in the weight department. But at some point, you will want to get very serious about weight loss and good nutrition. A registered dietitian is just the person who can help. These professionals have studied good nutrition and can save you time and experimentation on your own.

They are also good sources of inspiration and support. They are not weight-loss professionals, but weight control is at the core of what they do. A dietitian can help you understand why your food choices are not helping your cause, or perhaps are even hindering you in your mission to lose weight.

Your doctor should be able to direct you to some registered dietitians in your area. The local hospital will have a list of R.D.s. Many dietitians specialize in one area of health—cardiovascular, renal, and diabetes are common areas of specialization. Dietitians who specialize in diabetes may be right up your alley, if you and your endocrinologist have found that insulin resistance is at the core of your PCOS and weight issues.

What will a dietitian do? He or she will start by getting a personal history, asking questions about your past and your current eating habits, such as: "Have you always struggled with weight issues, or is this something new?" "What does a typical day look like for you, as far as meals and snacking are concerned?" "Do you eat out in restaurants a lot?" "Are you making meals for a family, or does someone else in your family do the cooking?" "What kind of work do you do?" "What do you do about lunch during the workday?" "Do you eat breakfast?"

The dietitian will then start to educate you on the basics of good nutrition and how it applies to your specific symptoms. He or she will then start to formulate an eating plan for you to lose, not gain, or to maintain your weight, whatever it is you are looking for.

Where to Begin?

If you are seriously obese, you will need to make drastic, immediate changes or be at risk for major and even life-threatening health concerns. However, if you are a few pounds overweight, it can be best to start with some small changes.

Those small changes can be with things that you do often, so they can add up to big results. Here are some possibilities:

Do you drink coffee with "extra cream"? Start mixing the cream with milk until, after a couple of weeks, you are using only milk, preferably low-fat milk. If you do that for a month or so, you will find cream in your coffee to be a bit repulsive! Better yet, work toward drinking coffee black, or not drinking coffee at all. Do you always drink tea black? Then try making the switch to tea altogether—not the solution if you want to get rid of caffeine, too, but if you are looking to lessen your fat intake, black tea or coffee is better than the beverage with cream or milk. Ditto with sugar in your coffee. Once you wean yourself from sugared coffee, if the server at your local coffee shop accidentally puts sugar in your coffee, you will notice immediately. You'll probably even go so far as to return it, since you'll find it so sweet as to be undrinkable!

Do you love potato chips or nachos, or other snack items? Don't try to give them up cold turkey and set yourself up to fail. Try instead to limit your consumption. If you normally grab the whole bag and sit in front of the television, or lie in the lawn chair reading a book and mindlessly reaching into the bag until it's empty, stop bringing the bag with you. Instead, take out a handful or perhaps the number of chips that is listed as a "serving size" on the nutrient chart. Seal the bag up, put it away, and enjoy your chips slowly. When your handful is gone, go find something to run off to do and keep yourself busy so the temptation to go back to the bag isn't there.

Don't let yourself get to the point of being extremely hungry. If you can, eat something light and nutritious or nonfattening every two to three hours. A piece of fruit is always good, or a small bowl of healthy cereal (not the sugar-coated kind) with low-fat milk, some yogurt, a handful of nuts. Then when you go to eat a main meal, you won't be so ravenous that you either pick things that are going to counteract your attempts to diet or devour a portion much larger than you really should or actually need.

Drink water. As mentioned above, there is debate at the moment about whether the old adage of eight glasses a day is really necessary. However, in addition to the evidence that consuming five or more eight-ounce glasses of water daily will reduce the risk of heart attacks, water is calorie-free and is required for your body to function and survive, making it always a good choice. Fruit juices are often full of sugar, real unsweetened fruit juices can be extremely expensive, diet sodas are full of chemicals—why not just go for water? Plus, a glass of water can help fill your stomach a bit and make you feel a little fuller before a meal, so you may be less tempted to eat more than an appropriate portion.

Change your "favorite" things. If you love ice cream and always have a bowl in the evening, don't give it up altogether and make yourself miserable. Instead, find a different favorite ice cream— look for a low-fat ice cream that you love, or find a frozen yogurt flavor that is delicious and eat that instead. And make your portion in line with the serving size on the package—even use a small bowl to force portion control. One of the common problems with low-fat food items is that people often think they can eat as much as you want, just because the item is low in fat. Some prepared low-fat foods are very high in sugar, something you want to cut back on when you are trying to lose weight.

Change some food-focused habits. Do you typically go out for pizza every Friday evening with your colleagues? Do they always want to order the Supreme pizza that has four different greasy meats on it and extra cheese? And you're always annoyed with yourself for eating twice as many slices as you want, because, after all, it tastes so good! And, of course, pizza often means beer. Try ordering your own personal-size pizza in a vegetarian version, no extra cheese, and eat just that small pizza. Better yet, eat just half of it, and bring the other half home for a quick lunch the next day on your busy Saturday. Skip the beer and order a diet soda or, better yet, a glass of water. If you don't feel you have the willpower to skip the beer or adjust your pizza intake, maybe for a while you should skip the Friday evening gathering altogether. Find a more healthful way to end the week, and make it your new routine.

Focus on your typical "food week," and come up with your own list of six to ten things that you could easily change to start to cut back on calories and fat.

Snacking Ideas

We have been conditioned to think snacking is bad, but, like everything else, it really just depends. Choosing the right snack items can actually help curb your appetite when mealtimes come, so you will more easily be able to stay within a good range of calorie intake at meals.

However, if you are counting calories and fat grams, don't forget to include your snack calories in your overall count—those couple of chocolate-coated graham crackers can add significant calories to your day. Here are some low-calorie and low-fat snacking ideas:

• Salsa with low-fat nacho chips or baked potato chips
• Pita bread with tabouli
• Unbuttered hot-air or microwave popcorn
• Granola bars
• Pretzels
• Fruit (but not late at night—fruit is high in fructose, which converts to energy if you are active, but if you eat it right before bedtime it will be converted immediately to fat)
• Vegetable wedges and no-fat sour cream or, better yet, salsa
• Frozen yogurt or low-fat ice cream
• Low-fat or fat-free yogurt. Add some frozen berries to add crunch and flavor without many calories.

As with everything you eat when it comes to losing weight, portion control is the key. A few nachos with no-fat salsa are a fine midafternoon snack; you just can't sit with the whole bag in front of you and snack until the jar of salsa is empty. Take a few chips out of the bag, seal it, and put it away. Dump a couple tablespoons of salsa into a small bowl. Eat your snack slowly and enjoy it. When that portion is done, you're done. If you are more than modestly overweight, it will probably be best to find a different dipper than nachos or even baked potato chips; try pretzels or crispy pita wedges.

Weight Control Franchises

Weight Watchers, Jenny Craig,® and other weight-loss franchises are all over the country. Strip malls nationwide host these businesses. You certainly do not need to join one in order to lose weight. However, for some women, the encouragement, motivation, and support are critical for weight-loss success. And the added discipline that comes from being weighed in once or twice a week is one more thing that will help them succeed.

Some of the franchises focus mainly on the support and motivation. You pay a membership fee that entitles you to chat with one of their consultants about your goals, sit in on membership meetings where you hear from other members about their successes and tips on subjects like eating out in restaurants, and you get menus and charts and other things to help make and measure progress toward your weight goals. Weight Watchers, for instance, usually has a couple of different weight-loss plans going at any one time, which allows you to choose the method that best suits your lifestyle, personality, and goals.

Other weight-loss franchises focus on selling prepared foods. These foods are specifically designed to help you meet calorie and fat intakes that you have worked out with the staff to meet your weight-loss goal. These types of programs can be expensive, but buying food and preparing meals for weight loss can be time-consuming. If you are either too busy or don't feel disciplined enough to spend the time in the grocery store and in front of the stove preparing meals, this type of program might be perfect for you. Don't forget, while the overall cost is sure to be higher, the money you spend on the diet program food is money you won't spend on other groceries.

Radical Weight-Loss Methods
Pills
In your effort to control your weight, you will run across many weight-loss claims that are attached to different kinds of pills. Many are too good to be true, and you will need to keep that old adage in mind: "If it's too good to be true, then it's probably not true." Drugs that are

marketed for weight loss represent a multibillion-dollar industry in America; it makes sense that companies would market them with the most appealing claims that they can.

Natural remedies are also prevalent for weight-control purposes. While many of these are useful and effective to some degree, do not take them to be completely harmless. Ephedra (derived from the herb ma huang) is a popular ingredient in over-the-counter weight-loss formulations. Ephedra has been known to cause fast/irregular heartbeats, angina, heart attacks, strokes, hypertension, urinary obstruction (in men with an enlarged prostate), anxiety, insomnia, and psychosis—hardly the profile of a harmless product! Since ephedra products are poorly regulated and not standardized, doses (and consequently side effects) can vary widely and unpredictably. The risk of side effects is increased even further if ephedra is combined with caffeine or any other stimulant. If you are taking medication, you should always consult with your physician, pharmacist, herbalist, or naturopath about the potential conflicts of the products.

Likewise, if you have existing health problems—some of them related to PCOS, some not—you need to be extremely cautious about anything you ingest. So-called "diet pills" are typically stimulants. The health effects on people with diseases and conditions such as diabetes, high blood pressure, cardiac disease, and even problems like insomnia can range from annoying to life-threatening.

So, the fact that you can walk into the drugstore or even the local convenience store and buy these products does not mean they are innocuous. Prescription appetite suppressants may be helpful in some situations, but these medicines are not totally benign either (which is why they require a prescription). The best way to lose weight is still to gain control of your eating habits and increase the amount of exercise you get.

Surgical Options

Bariatric surgery, controlling weight by surgery, is a very radical form of weight control that is becoming more popular. There are several different avenues that this form of weight control takes, but the basic aim is to change the way your stomach receives food. One method is to reduce the actual size of the stomach so you feel full faster. Another is to bypass part of the intestine.

Other surgical interventions are to wire the jaw so that the person can only take in small amounts of food, or even only food in the form of liquid.

These kinds of surgery have become regular topics on the evening network news. Although you will hear and read about these methods, they are drastic indeed and are really intended for the severely overweight individual who has no other recourse. Surgery is not a necessary route for the PCOS patient. There are so many other factors to gain control of, some of which will most likely help with weight control, that PCOS women would have to be extremely obese, have exhausted every other option, and have serious long-lasting health implications to make surgery a wise option.

The Psychological Component

Controlling the weight issues that are problematic for PCOS patients can be broken down into four elements:

1. Everyday eating and nutrition
2. Dieting to lose weight
3. The psychological component
4. Exercise

All four are critical to dealing with weight.

Most syndromes like PCOS have a catch-22 that has to be dealt with. In this case it is the fact that PCOS sufferers, because of hormonal and other biological issues brought on by the condition, are prone to weight gain and obesity. However, it is clear that losing weight has immediate positive effects on combating PCOS.

We've covered the good nutrition and dieting aspect of weight control. We will cover exercise in the next chapter. Let's spend a little time on the psychological and emotional component of weight control.

Sources of Motivation, Support, and Discipline for Weight-Loss Success
Losing weight is a difficult proposition under any circumstances. The roller-coaster ride that PCOS takes you on adds another whole dimension to dieting stress. There are many ways you can combat the stress of a weight-loss program, motivate yourself to begin, and stay motivated amidst some difficult odds for long-term success. Here are some ideas:

1. Learn all you can about the significant benefits PCOS patients experience from weight loss. Knowledge can be a major motivator. Any time you get exasperated with your diet, thinking of these benefits can keep you going.

2. Once you've been dieting for a bit and have begun to lose some weight, and you have experienced some of the aforementioned benefits, this alone may be one of the strongest motivating factors. Slipping into a size smaller pair of pants, reclaiming some of those favorite items in the back of your closet, and soaking up those comments from your friends can be the best motivation you can get.

3. Get some outside support. Diet with a friend—you can keep each other on track, share dieting tips, and share great diet

foods and recipes. Hospitals are becoming major outlets for information, holding seminars and clinics given by professionals. Check your local hospital for possible programs on weight loss and weight control. Organized, commercial weight-loss programs such as Weight Watchers and Jenny Craig are good motivators in this regard as well.

4. Do it for yourself. Don't look at thin models and slim movie stars and put pressure on yourself to look like them, in order to fit into some artificial measure of beauty. Many of them fully admit that they don't even look like themselves first thing in the morning! While your husband or partner will probably be the first to compliment you as you lose weight (and women who take off a few pounds often motivate overweight partners to do the same!), it is limiting and can be self-defeating to lose weight because someone else thinks you should look different. Do it for yourself first—for your overall health, to alleviate your PCOS symptoms, to more easily do an activity that you like to do, and to feel better from your own reflection in the mirror, too!

5. Set realistic goals. Losing weight takes time. Not only are those "lose ten pounds in two days" ads false, but that kind of weight loss is unhealthy. Plan to lose maybe three to five pounds a month for six months to a year. Give yourself time to adjust to a new way of eating—which is the key to ongoing weight control, once you've lost weight—and to incorporating more exercise into your life.

6. If you go off your diet and new eating habits for an evening or even a weekend, don't despair, and most of all don't quit! Just pick up where you left off and forget about the digression.

7. Find ways to reward yourself. Keep it simple—don't create rewards that make you feel guilty. If you are struggling with finances, don't reward yourself with expensive purchases. But if you meet a major weight goal, maybe a new scarf or a pair of earrings is a satisfying reward. If you love real ice cream, treat yourself at the local ice cream shop—but get a kid-size portion of something simple, not a huge banana split for which you are suddenly going to feel guilty. You need to celebrate!

8. Don't weigh yourself every day. This can be very discouraging, since our body weight can fluctuate by two to three pounds per day from simple water retention, without our doing much of anything different. Instead, pick two or three days a week to weigh in, say Friday and Monday. Give yourself a range—I'd like to stay within 155-160 pounds for the next couple of weeks. During those couple of weeks, look for ways in your eating and exercise program to drop to the next level. Then spend a couple of weeks holding under 155.

If a special event comes up and you suspect you will go off your diet over the weekend, you will feel better if you are within your range on Friday. Then if Monday's weigh-in shows that you splurged enough to go above your desired range, you have the whole week to get back on track from there and compare again on Friday.

Weight loss is difficult enough. Don't put additional stress on yourself. Instead spend your energy motivating yourself, shopping for new clothes, and figuring out what you are going to do with the extra time from going to fewer doctors' appointments, since you will almost certainly have fewer symptoms to deal with!

A PERSONAL STORY

Carol

In her early teens, Carol and her doctor dismissed her irregular periods as nothing to be concerned over, just the normal "settling in" of her cycle. "Being young," Carol said, "you really don't analyze it much." Her doctor assured her that sometimes it takes a while for your body to work it out, and her periods would certainly normalize as she got older. They never did.

Not only that, but she experienced more than her fair share of acne problems. And she couldn't understand the excessive facial hair she had. Not extreme, but different enough from her friends to make her self-conscious about it.

Even dealing with all these things was minor compared to the key issue for Carol—trying to control her weight. No small issue for a young woman who'd been training to be a competitive figure skater from the age of ten.

Her doctors told her she needed to lose weight, but she couldn't understand how she could still be overweight when she hardly ate anything. She had been raised a vegetarian and continued to be one. And she was far from a couch potato—her skating schedule was demanding, with training starting before school each morning and continuing for four, and sometimes five, more hours after school as well. The pressure was intense.

"My coaches and choreographers were telling me to be thin, and my sponsors and my parents were investing so much in me," Carol said. Her solution was to turn to eating disorders. By age fourteen, Carol was anorexic and bulimic, and she got down to 100 pounds.

Carol gave up the competitive skating late in her high-school years. Her weight crept up and, by her early twenties, Carol had solved her eating disorders and gained over 100 pounds. Shortly after she started gaining weight, her periods stopped altogether. For a while, this didn't seem like a bad thing—not dealing with the monthly issue of having your period has its appeal! But after a while, Carol concluded it was not normal and probably not good for her.

Finally, a little over one year ago, at age thirty-one, Carol began to see a doctor at a clinic in Boston that combines Chinese and Western medicine. During the first visit, after she described her history, Carol's doctor mentioned polycystic ovarian syndrome. When Carol got home, she almost immediately began researching PCOS, something she had never heard of. She began to read the reports from women about the symptoms they had and the issues they dealt with. Carol could not believe it. "These women were me," she said. They were all telling her story.

Things started to tumble much more into place after that first visit. During her second visit, the doctor lined her up for some blood work, but not enough for Carol. The research she had read suggested much more extensive blood work than her doctor was calling for. She insisted they have the extra testing done. Her insulin level was very high, suggesting hyperinsulinemia, a major culprit in PCOS, according to the research she had read. She was diagnosed with insulin resistance. Carol then went to a reproductive endocrinologist, following up on that hormone connection that was prevalent in her reading.

When Carol asked her doctor about checking her ovaries for the classic cysts, her doctor insisted her ovaries were fine. But how could he be so sure? It was just his feeling, he said. Carol again got assertive and insisted on an ultrasound to check them for certain, and tried to push for a vaginal ultrasound, which would give a more accurate view. The doctor finally agreed to the more basic exterior ultrasound. When Carol went for the appointment, she ended up having the vaginal ultrasound after all. And it showed that her ovaries were covered with cysts.

But still the most frustrating issue for Carol was the inability to get her weight under control. As she gained weight, the other symptoms grew worse, a vicious cycle that Carol was desperate to break. Her doctor recommended she concentrate on diet and exercise and that she see a nutritionist to help. Carol was open to any possibilities, and began once a month to see a dietician who works with PCOS patients. As she got into a good diet and exercise plan, her monthly visits began to taper off to more occasional visits. And her weight began to taper off as well.

The dietician put Carol on a 40-30-30 diet (40 percent carbohydrate/30 percent protein/30 percent fat), sort of a simplified "Zone Diet." Carol has lost forty pounds since working with the dietician. Getting in that 30 percent protein has been difficult for a vegetarian—especially since she needs to avoid tofu, often a major protein source for vegetarians, but also a food high in the hormone estrogen—but she's been able to make it work. She also went on a vitamin regimen and uses some herbs, such as saw palmetto, which is used to regulate male hormones. She has chosen to stay away from prescribed medication for now and prefers to go the nutrition route and know that the drugs are there if she's stuck.

The good news? Just two weeks after starting the diet and exercise program, she got her first period in two years!

Carol's advice to other women sorting through the complexities of PCOS comes direct from her own experience: "You need to think about yourself and be aggressive in getting what you feel you need out of the medical system. If I hadn't been so assertive, then I wouldn't be where I am now. Do it for yourself, focus on yourself."

CHAPTER SEVEN ∽

The Second Important Step to PCOS Control
Exercise

Creating a diet and establishing new eating habits are the first key to losing weight. These two things alone can take you a significant way toward getting to the weight you would like to see when you step on the scale. However, the addition of exercise to any weight-loss program is critical for the next level of weight loss and for ongoing success in keeping weight off.

The benefits of weight control for the PCOS patient cannot be stressed too much. To be serious about controlling PCOS, instead of being controlled by it, means being serious about weight loss and weight control—unless of course you are among the minority of women with PCOS for whom weight is not a problem. Chances are great, however, that if you have been diagnosed with PCOS, being overweight is high on your list of symptoms.

Working with the diet and nutrition suggestions in the last chapter—including incorporating a dietitian into your health team—will take you far. Once you really get portion control, nutritional balance, and good snacking habits under way, combined with understanding how the food you eat affects your body and therefore your PCOS symptoms, you will see significant weight loss.

But once that first significant loss is experienced, you will almost invariably hit a plateau. If you and your doctor have determined that you need to lose twenty-five pounds, you may lose that first fifteen pounds just by these dietary changes alone! But the last ten pounds will probably come a little harder. And that's a key place where exercise fits in.

PCOS Does Make It Harder

A woman with PCOS has a much harder time losing weight than she would if she did not have the syndrome. The hormonal factors are such a significant player that weight loss can be frustrating at best. It's hard not to just give up and decide that, because of your condition, there is no way you are going to lose weight—but don't give up! If you tackle both the underlying causes and the overweight issues, you will see positive effects. You may just have to be more patient than most.

Nutritional changes and classic dieting are the first steps to weight loss, especially for PCOS patients. However, incorporating a logical, relatively vigorous exercise regimen is going to make a difference, help you lose weight, and make you feel better. Just when you feel that it's hopeless and think about quitting your diet and exercise plan, you could be on the brink of major changes. There are some ways to encourage yourself to believe in a positive outcome.

Don't Do Everything at Once

If you have been tackling your diet but haven't incorporated an exercise program into your routine yet, don't beat yourself up. You can only deal with so many things at a time! Changing your diet and adding organized exercise to your day are huge efforts and often require a completely new outlook. No one can change these things all at once. If you try, you will probably give up too soon. Take things in increments and add to your PCOS management program when the last stage has become second nature. PCOS didn't creep up on you last night—you don't need to change everything today.

Motivation

If you concentrate your time at first on losing weight and get that significant weight-loss period established, that will propel you to the benefits of exercising. Imagine the motivating factor of losing ten or fifteen pounds! And once you lose this amount of weight, the chances are good that other PCOS-related symptoms will start to subside as well. Studies have shown that only a 5 percent reduction in weight—that's eight pounds for a 160-pound woman—can have a significant impact on reducing symptoms and regulating menstrual cycles. Make use of any weight-loss momentum and start to work on the exercise component of weight loss.

Some women with PCOS, unfortunately, have a much more difficult time losing weight. In these cases, it is best to get the dietary changes, weight-loss plans, and the exercise program under way all at once. However, that still doesn't mean you need to slam dunk yourself with huge changes to your diet and huge additions to your daily exercise. Add new pieces to the weight-loss puzzle in increments you can handle.

Perhaps you are one of those people who, when you decide to do something, go for the gusto. Good for you! Here's a place where that attitude is going to serve you well. Just make sure you aren't one of the millions who go for gusto and then find that the gusto disappears in a short period of time. Women with PCOS need to be in it for the long haul. Marathon runners train differently than sprinters—you need to approach your plan differently than for a short-term venture as well.

Where Do I Begin?

The first place to start with any exercise program is with your doctor. Be sure that you know what your overall health risks are, and pick suitable exercise outlets to meet any limitations you may have. As you exercise and lose weight, your health risks will probably diminish, and you can always talk with your doctor about adding new activities at that point.

A common pitfall for people who find themselves needing to become more physically fit is this: I need to lose weight, I need to get more fit, so I will join the local fitness center and spend two hours, four days a week, and do weight lifting, use the treadmill, swim, and join the aerobics class—that should do it.

That should do it all right—what it will do is last about two to three weeks before the novelty wears off and you realize that there is just no way you can fit that kind of exercise into your week's schedule. Even if you have all the time in the world, someone who has not already been motivated to create a formal exercise program for herself is not suddenly going to become that interested.

Don't set yourself up to fail. Just start slowly with a couple things that can make a difference. Start by deciding you will do something specifically active three days each week.

Some Simple Ideas

Here's a list of ideas for beginning to incorporate exercise into your life. Some of these you have heard a million times, read in a magazine, seen on the wall of the doctor's office. But they are a way to get started.

- Find a way to incorporate brisk walking into your day. Park in a faraway spot in the office parking lot. If you don't have a dog, walk the neighbor's dog two or three times a week. Walk around the mall three times a week—chances are you need to shop for something at least one of those times anyway. And, yes, take the stairs instead of the elevator.

- Join an organized sports team. If there isn't one in your area, consider starting one—that can be a good way to make sure it is noncompetitive, just a fun game intended for some exercise. Choose something that is within your current level of fitness: an easy softball game, tennis match, basketball, bowling. If you are not accustomed to exercising, at this point anything that gets you up and moving around is good, even if it's just once a week on Saturday mornings or Wednesday evenings.

- The idea of getting to a fitness center can be daunting to women with kids. If there is any way possible, carve out an area in your home to put a treadmill or an exercise bicycle. These activities can be boring, so find ways to make them interesting. Buy some great mystery books or fun magazines and keep them with the exercise machine—make it a rule that you can only read them while you are exercising. A good Rita Mae Brown or Robert Parker mystery will get you back to the machine on a regular basis!

- Speaking of kids, having children in the home is often the first excuse women use to have no time to exercise. Incorporate the kids into your exercise program! Volunteer to be a coach. Organize a mother/child softball, soccer, or volleyball team. Use your kids to get you out and exercising instead of using them as an excuse not to.

• Keep a basketball hoop, soccer goal, or volleyball net in the backyard. Have your own little pickup basketball games with your kids or your husband or partner or the next-door neighbor. Sweat a little!

• Once or twice a month, go on one of those walks-for-a-cause. There is one going on near you almost every weekend of the year. Take one of the kids with you, ask your partner to go along. Exercise for two causes: for a nonprofit organization and for yourself! And you will find yourself walking to "train" whenever a walkathon is coming up.

• Get a few free weights for home. These are not going to do much for weight loss, but shaping and toning can become very motivating once you've begun to lose weight through diet and aerobic exercises. Don't overwhelm yourself and go out and immediately buy a weight bench, bars, and several hundred pounds of weights. Just get a couple of five-pound weights and work specifically on your arms. Stick with a couple of weight-lifting exercises three times a week for two to three months. You will be surprised what it does to tone your arms—then you'll be motivated for more!

Many people dive right in full force. Instead of being motivated for more, they burn themselves out within three weeks to a month. Be realistic but don't procrastinate—get started, even with the smallest exercise plan.

Fitting It In

Your first thought will be that there is no way you will be able to fit exercising into your day. You have kids, you have a stressful job, or even both.

If you are motivated enough to keep control of your weight and get beyond that plateau of your early weight loss from diet changes, *you absolutely can fit some level of exercise into your day.* You will need to be creative with ideas like those above, and you need to have motivation—the latter you will hopefully be getting from your strides toward losing weight.

Once you begin to get into exercise, you will find the time no matter what. The exercise outlet that you choose will become such an important part of your day that you will find ways to fit it in. And once you really begin to see the benefits, wild horses won't stop you!

Getting Serious

You lost ten pounds after three or four months on your new eating plan. You started to incorporate some consistent but low-level exercise and noticed you're slimmer and looking more toned. Not anything hugely significant yet, but definitely noticeable. Let the motivation take over! You are poised at this moment to really begin to make exercise an important part of your life. Now is the time to expect a little more from yourself, to pull in some of the more time-consuming types of exercise and exercise programs.

Personal Trainers

If you think you don't have time to exercise regularly, you certainly don't have time to plan your own exercise program. Consider signing on with a personal trainer (PT). Personal trainers:

- Know a lot about nutrition and dieting, and will and help you learn about your own body mass index and other useful diagnostic tools for weight control.

- Will teach you how to use exercise equipment—including free weights—most effectively for what you are trying to accomplish, efficiently for your needs, and safely so you don't give yourself medical problems with strains and unnecessarily sore muscles.

- Set up an exercise program for you to follow.

- Are great motivators! Because their work depends on their clients continuing to work with them, it is to their benefit that you follow through with an exercise program and see results, so you'll be motivated to continue.

If cost is a factor, find a personal trainer to work with who will consider meeting with you just once a month. A concentrated amount of time at first is best so you can get lots of input on what you are doing. After that, you can maintain a certain level for a month, then check in with your PT to make sure you are on track for your goals and to take you to the next level.

Your local YMCA/YWCA or other fitness center will have personal trainers who use their facilities. Some work from their own space. If cost is not a factor, there are personal trainers who do home visits! Some of them can even bring equipment with them. Or, if you want to work with a PT at home, he or she can help you purchase the right equipment for your needs and for the amount of space you have to devote to exercise equipment.

Decide on a personal trainer just as you would establish any other professional relationship—only more so. In order to get the help you need, you must be very comfortable with your PT and talk with her or him honestly and straightforwardly. You can't hide the fact that you have gone off your diet since you saw your PT a month ago. You are the one who is getting the real benefit from this relationship, so you need to be upfront with your trainer.

As with any aspect of exercise that is new to you, be sure to talk with your doctor before starting to work with a personal trainer. A professional PT will have health documents you need to sign and have your doctor sign as well. You will also be asked to make out a complete health and fitness history on yourself. Definitely tell your PT about your PCOS diagnosis so he or she can tailor your program wtih that in mind.

What Can I Do on My Own?

Besides the day-to-day things mentioned in the previous list, what are some things you can do to get started on a serious exercise regimen? If you are more than a few pounds overweight, start off with something that will get your body more flexible and more in tune with the idea of exercising. Plus, they are all great stress-reducers—and most women trying to manage PCOS can use some help reducing stress. Some ideas are:

> *Tai chi:* Tai chi is a martial art that uses slow, calculated movements to increase balance, flexibility, and awareness. Tai chi can help calm you and get you in touch with your body. It is sort of like meditation in motion. Many fitness centers and wellness centers offer tai chi classes. Tai chi is also something that can be fairly easy to learn and follow from a video—you can do it in the comfort of your living room, wearing baggy pants and an oversized t-shirt.

Yoga: Don't consider yoga as something only for thin, extremely flexible people. Yoga is great for everyone—and the more yoga you do, the more you can do! If you don't consider yourself very flexible, or tend to be self-conscious about doing things like yoga in a group, you can get videos and do yoga at home. It doesn't take any special equipment, although it can be helpful to have someone assessing the accuracy of your positions—some yoga requires very specific body position in order to avoid injury. Once you get into yoga, you will look forward to your sessions. And after you've grown accustomed to some of the positions and moves, consider tapes that are directed toward using yoga for weight loss. These sessions move along quickly—you don't even realize what a workout you've had until you're done!

Swimming: If you have the time and access to a good pool, swimming can be a great form of exercise. The water allows you to exercise rigorously with less impact on your body than exercise out of water.

Simple exercises: Some exercises take no equipment at all. Start by fitting in three sets of eight or ten abdominal crunches, three times a week. This will take no more than ten minutes, max. After a couple of weeks, when you begin to feel as if you aren't doing much of anything, add two or four reps to each set. That's already as much as thirty-six crunches three times a week! Now you are getting somewhere. Gradually add a few other things such as leg lifts or push-ups. If you don't think you have the time for this, plan to do it every Monday, Wednesday, and Friday before you shower. On those days, reduce your showering time—instead of a luxurious shower, wash up quickly, and maybe just lather your hair and rinse, but don't "repeat" as the shampoo bottle says to do. Get a shampoo that includes conditioner so you only have to rinse your hair once. Use these extra minutes for another set of abdominal crunches.

Sex: It had to be mentioned. Perhaps your PCOS symptoms make sex seem an unattractive activity at the moment. If you have a committed relationship and wish sex were not so complicated by your PCOS symptoms, take a little extra time to make yourself feel like being intimate, and use the additional motivation that lovemaking is excellent exercise!

Stepping It Up a Notch

After a month or two of getting your body used to the idea of exercising, when your day doesn't seem complete without some form of exercise, you can start to pick up the pace a little. Now is the time to have some additional expectations of yourself. This is the period when you will begin to see, if you are diligent, some real steps forward in your weight loss, and some real notches backward on the scale!

Here are some ideas for picking up the pace without going overboard:

Weight-training: The machines at the fitness center are designed to put you in the proper position for lifting weights and for doing a circuit that hits all muscle groups in your body. If you have started doing free-weight training on a modest level at home and find you like it, you will love the weight machines. Either a staff member at the fitness center or your personal trainer if you have one should walk you through the machines the first time. They will point out important safety issues, show you how to properly sit in the machine, explain how to change weight amounts, and give you a recommendation for the number of repetitions and sets you might want to start with. Schedule a little extra time for this first visit, and learn how to properly use the machines. By the time you do the full circuit, you will definitely feel that you have had a workout! Do this circuit diligently three times a week for three months, and you will definitely see some changes in your body!

Squash, racquetball, or handball: If you are the competitive type, a rousing game of racquetball can give you quite a workout. You and your game partner can choose the pace; you may find that you have so much fun you aren't even thinking about the fact that you are exercising!

Aerobics workout: As with yoga and tai chi, many fitness and wellness centers offer aerobics classes. You can start out with a low-impact aerobics program and move up to a more rigorous program once you get into it. If you don't like the idea of bouncing around in a group, there are many videos and even television programs devoted to a daily workout that you can do in the privacy of your own living room.

Things to Remember While Exercising

If regular exercise has not been part of your life before now, there are some important points to keep in mind while you exercise:

- For any vigorous workout, drink plenty of fluids. Water is always best.

- The claim that stretching is crucial has come under scrutiny, but the jury is still out, so stretch both before and after your workout. Even if further study proves that its benefits have been exaggerated, gentle stretching probably can never be bad.

- Don't overwhelm and discourage yourself, and don't choose to get your exercise doing something you simply don't like to do. It's OK not to like to swim or lift weights or whatever. In order to be successful and be motivated to continue, you need to choose an exercise regimen you don't hate.

• The old adage "no pain, no gain" is not true. You should not be in pain either during exercise or after. You may feel some discomfort the next day, but your muscles should not hurt.

• When lifting weights, start off with a low weight size. You can always increase it, if it seems way too easy, but don't decide that until you've done several repetitions in a few sets. The idea is to have the last few repetitions be a little strenuous, so if you pick up a weight and it seems too light, give it a whirl with three sets of a dozen repetitions before you decide to move up in weight. You might be surprised how tough those last few reps are. You don't want to sideline yourself from the start by straining muscles. Gradual buildup is the name of the exercise game. And always give yourself one day of rest between weight-lifting rounds.

• Mix it up. You don't have to get all your exercise from one activity. Some exercise regimes, such as weight lifting, do require repeating at least twice a week to make any progress at all, however slow. But if you just want to get some aerobic exercise, do some strenuous walking, ride a bicycle—mobile or stationary—take an aerobics class all in one week! And top it off by going dancing on Saturday night.

• Learn good posture. Not just your daily posture for sitting and standing and working at the computer, but the proper posture for the exercise you have chosen.

• Learn good breathing techniques. Most people pay little attention to their breathing, but breathing is critical for exercising well. Practicing deep, rhythmic breathing during the course of the day can even be a great stress reliever. Slowly take air into your abdomen first, fill up your mid-chest section, and then your upper chest/lungs. Exhale in the opposite way. Good breathing is simply good for you, but it is crucial while exercising.

The Ultimate Motivation

As mentioned earlier, beginning to lose weight and beginning to feel fit are extremely good motivators in their own right. The other important thing to understand is the chemical reactions taking place in your body as you exercise, lose weight, and gain fitness.

Body-fat levels trigger hormonal reactions. This is seen early in a girl's life when body fat ratio essentially tells the reproductive system that the physical body is now mature enough to begin reproductive life. This message is given via the hormones.

Body-fat levels continue throughout your life to trigger hormones in the body. As we now know with PCOS, your body's production and use of insulin is the key factor, typically an inability to use the insulin that the pancreas generates. This causes a condition known as hyper-insulinemia—elevated levels of insulin in the bloodstream. Even though there is plenty of insulin in the body, insulin resistance prevents the cells from using it, so the pancreas continues to get the message from the cells that they need insulin. The pancreas complies until either there is enough insulin that cells use at least some of it, or the pancreas says, "Whoa, this is all the insulin I can produce," and gives up in exhaustion.

In this hyperinsulinemic state, the ovaries get the message to step up testosterone production. Testosterone is, as we know, an androgen—one of the male hormones. More testosterone means male hair growth.

Ah, the connection is coming clear—more body fat means more insulin, which means an abnormal level of testosterone, which, in a woman, means annoying, visible, and often embarrassing symptoms.

Yes, gaining fitness and reducing body fat can mean fairly immediate reduction in symptoms related to testosterone levels, such as acne and hirsutism. For the woman who suffers dramatically from these symptoms, reducing these symptoms alone can be enough to keep her motivated to exercise and manage her diet.

A Final Word

Finally, don't beat yourself up if you miss an exercise session, or you don't feel you are losing weight fast enough, or you are starting off with a very low-level fitness program. Always keep in mind that PCOS is a chronic condition unique to each woman who has it, and you have the rest of your life to figure out what works for you and what doesn't. Instead, pat yourself on the back for simply getting started!

A PERSONAL STORY

Susan

Susan and her husband had been trying to conceive for six months. At twenty-eight years old, Susan wanted to get her family started and decided she wasn't willing to give it another six months. She had menstrual cycles, but her tracking of them showed that they were irregular, making timing conception difficult.

When she walked into her appointment with her obstetrician, Susan handed her doctor a list of various symptoms she was experiencing. Without hesitation, her doctor said "Oh, PCOS."

The symptoms Susan was having were mild but classic PCOS symptoms: mood swings, irritability, weight-control issues, and some excessive hair growth. But her primary concern was the inability to get pregnant. With that in mind, she got an ovulation detector kit and found that, in fact, she was not ovulating with every cycle. Her doctor prescribed an ovulation-stimulating drug called Clomid. Within three months, Susan was pregnant.

A little less than two years after her first child was born, Susan got pregnant again, and this time it was a "spontaneous pregnancy"—no assistance needed. And this time she had twins. Her PCOS symptoms, she says, were reduced when she was pregnant, and this carried through the whole time she was nursing her children.

Her twins are over three years old now, and Susan's PCOS symptoms are back. However, they are still minor and, with three young children—two still preschoolers—Susan does not have the amount of time it might take to work with an endocrinologist and other specialists to figure out how to control the underlying hormonal imbalances that may be at the root of her weight gain and hair growth. Susan suspects that the root cause of her PCOS may also be the cause of the anxiety she now controls through medication—both of which, the anxiety itself and the medications to control it, have their own side effects.

One aspect of PCOS that is currently frustrating Susan is that she never knows when her period will start. This makes birth control a bit of a challenge. She has tried birth-control pills in the past, but was just not able to get into the routine of taking them every day, and the pill made her gain weight, an issue that most women with PCOS already have to deal with.

For now, with just mild minor symptoms and her family established, fertility is no longer an issue for Susan, and she can cope with the symptoms she has. Her career in library science and her natural ability as a researcher help her keep tabs on advances in PCOS knowledge and treatment options, via the Internet and through the experiences of other PCOS women she sees regularly in her "twins club."

CHAPTER EIGHT ∽

Fertility

You may have opened this book and turned to this chapter first. With perhaps menstrual irregularity in teenage girls running a close second, fertility problems are the main reasons that many women end up in an endocrinologist's office and are subsequently diagnosed with PCOS.

If you have few or no monthly periods, you simply won't get pregnant. The natural processes that your body is designed to undergo, to allow an egg to be fertilized and to sustain pregnancy, as described in Chapter Two, are just not happening. Without an egg in the proper place to receive a sperm, conception does not take place. Without ovulation, an egg will not be in the proper place to receive the sperm. And even if all that happens, the incidence of miscarriage for women with PCOS is thought to be higher than average—the body's environment is not conducive to sustaining pregnancy.

But don't despair! May women with PCOS become pregnant readily, once they get some key symptoms under control. And many times these pregnancies occur without fertility intervention.

The Good News

As we've said many times throughout this book, there is a good news side to your problems with infertility—if that is what got you to the point of being diagnosed, you are at the beginning of the journey to having PCOS symptoms take a backseat in your life. With a diagnosis, you, not PCOS, can start to sort out how to be the driver of your hormonal life.

If PCOS is causing hyperinsulinemia, excess androgen load, or other hormone imbalances, getting to the root cause of hormonal imbalances in your endocrine system will quite likely be the turning point for fertility. Your hormones work to pave the roads and put up the signal lights to let your reproductive system perform the way it needs to, in order for you to get pregnant.

A Word of Caution

The chances that a PCOS diagnosis and resulting treatment will have positive results on your ability to get pregnant are very high. However, you cannot assume that PCOS and its symptoms are the sole reason for infertility. Infertility is a complex issue, with not only dozens of possible causes but also the complicating factor that two people—a man and woman—with very different hormonal and reproductive processes are crucial players. A woman's egg can make all the right moves and be ready for fertilization, but that is not going to happen without a vibrant sperm that manages to make the entire precarious journey.

A lot of times how you proceed depends on your age. If you are in your mid-twenties and can't get pregnant, you can afford to take the time to check into the "easiest" possible causes of infertility and work your way through them, one at a time, until you find the one that is preventing you from conceiving. However, if you are in your late thirties and trying to get pregnant, you may want to tackle a few possible causes for infertility at the same time.

A PCOS diagnosis is always a possible culprit for infertility. However, it is not always the cause. So if you are nearing the end of your reproductive years, it is not in your best interest to focus solely on PCOS as the cause of your specific infertility problems. By no means ignore the PCOS! But while you are working on regulating your hormones, you can also be checked for other possible causes—and your partner should be checked for possible infertility issues as well.

It is really up to you whether you take a step-by-step, one-thing-at-a-time approach or whether you take a multilevel approach. Whatever you decide, be sure to consult with your primary care doctor, OB/GYN, endocrinologist, and any other specialist you may be seeing. Weigh all the input that you get, then decide with your partner how best to proceed.

If you tackle your PCOS symptoms and start to see changes—regular periods, weight loss, and other symptoms subsiding—but you still aren't getting pregnant, it definitely is time to consider other infertility factors.

Addressing a PCOS diagnosis is certainly a legitimate place to start and may be the thing that sets the pregnancy ball in motion, but don't be too depressed if it doesn't turn out to be the only issue. Even if other things are involved in infertility, you will almost certainly be ahead of the game by getting your PCOS symptoms in check anyway.

The couple experiencing an inability to conceive will need to do some high-level investigating into their entire lifestyle, diet, exercise, physical health, and mental health. Your mental, or emotional, health can play a huge factor in fertility. Fertility problems are categorized in many areas, from anovulation to endometriosis to PCOS to male-related issues, but a large number are categorized as "unexplainable."

Don't be too quick to accept that! In some instances, "unexplainable" can be the doctor's excuse for not doing further testing—it all depends on how deeply you want to explore the matter. And when it comes to fertility, many couples want to explore the issue quite extensively.

All of this serves to emphasize the fact that being aware of and proactive about your health is a smart thing to do—if you practice good nutrition, exercise moderately, and pay attention to your health in general, you will be many steps ahead in the fertility game when you decide to try to get pregnant. Even if you still experience infertility, if you are within your healthy weight range, eat right, and keep fit, you will not have to work on those three areas of your lifestyle but can get right down to other possible problems.

The One-Year Rule of Thumb

A fertility rule of thumb is to try to get pregnant for a year. There are so many factors that need to fall into place—sometimes the stress of trying to get pregnant itself can lead to infertility—that one year seems to be a good amount of time to determine whether all the right factors simply need to naturally fall into place. If you do not get pregnant within that one-year period, then you have fertility problems.

If you have perfectly regular periods, are within the optimum weight range for your height and body type, eat well, exercise regularly, and are in general good health, then perhaps trying for a year is an appropriate choice. But if you do not cycle regularly, simply trying to get pregnant for a year is probably just going to put you a year behind. And again, if you are over thirty-five years old, playing the one-year game may not be the most logical choice.

It would seem logical to say that if you have any signs of the PCOS symptoms that you have read about throughout this book, then a visit to a fertility clinic is recommended. However, keep in mind the diverse nature of PCOS symptoms—some of the symptoms are conditions you may not suspect to be signs of PCOS or infertility. How likely is one to think of acne being at all related to an inability to get pregnant?

How PCOS Symptoms Affect Fertility
The Hormone Factor
PCOS has pretty much been determined to be a problem of the endocrine system, despite the fact that many women come to a diagnosis through the fertility clinic. Hormones play a huge role in pregnancy—in a way, the hormonal role in pregnancy is like the role of fuel in driving a car. You can play around with the instruments—move the steering wheel, blink the lights, play the radio—but, without gas in the tank, you won't get to where you want to go. Without proper hormonal influence, you will not get pregnant.

As you know from preceding chapters, glucose impairment and insulin resistance are two of the many PCOS side effects. Both are concerned with how the body processes nutrition. If the body is insulin resistant—that is, is not responding adequately to the insulin being produced by the pancreas—then the pancreas will pump out more in an attempt to get its message across. The body then experiences an abnormal spike in the insulin level in the bloodstream, which in turns gives signals to other hormones.

The key signal that relates to fertility is the message to the ovaries to boost production of androgen (those pesky male hormones that even women have). This high level of male hormones in the system results in the ovary not releasing an egg. The developing follicles that don't ultimately release an egg are the cysts seen on the ultrasound of a typical PCOS patient.

And a sperm can swim its little heart out, but if it never finds an egg to fertilize, there is no pregnancy.

The Weight Factor

Obesity prevalence in PCOS is a double-edged sword. How the body is processing glucose (or, more accurately, not processing it) adds to the propensity toward obesity in women with PCOS. Obesity, according to the Mayo Clinic Web site, worsens the body's insulin resistance. This, in turn, increases the androgen and insulin levels in the bloodstream. All of which has a huge impact on whether or not you get pregnant.

Sometimes, women with PCOS find that they become pregnant shortly after reducing their weight.

What If I'm Not Overweight?

Although women with PCOS predominantly are overweight to varying degrees, not all PCOS patients are overweight. Women who are thin can be insulin resistant and have PCOS and even diabetes. Weight loss has such a dramatic and rapid impact in alleviating PCOS symptoms that thin women may have a little more difficulty addressing symptoms—diet and exercise may help some, but they may find that they have to resort to medical treatments to see strong results. Or they may find that they have no difficulty getting pregnant, or become pregnant with very minor types of intervention, such as a few months on metformin.

Surgical Treatments

There are a few surgical treatments that are performed on women with PCOS, especially if they are trying to get pregnant. However, the recommendation consistently is that these should be attempted only after other less invasive medical treatments have been tried without success. Before the hormone connection was made, these surgeries were among the limited treatment options. Two such procedures are:

> *Laparoscopic ovarian drilling (also known as ovarian diathermy treatment):* Usually a procedure tried only after drug therapies have not produced the desired results, laparoscopic ovarian drilling is done via a tube with a camera inserted through an incision in the abdomen. Enlarged follicles on the ovaries are burned using laser or electrical energy. According to the Mayo Clinic Web site, "The goal is to reduce levels of LH and androgen hormones. Doctors aren't sure how this occurs. One theory is that drilling destroys hormone-producing ovarian cells." Although laparoscopic ovarian drilling is still very much done with caution, one study at the Royal Victorian Hospital at McGill University in Montreal, Canada, shows that it can be helpful in women who are Clomiphene-resistant. The procedure was shown to increase ovulation in 70-90 percent of patients, and produce pregnancy rates of 70 percent, although some reports have shown a wide range of pregnancy results as well.

> The thinking is that reducing the amount of hormone-producing tissue area (i.e., the ovary) with these procedures will allow the endocrine system to work better in that tissue.

> *Ovarian wedge resection:* Just as the name implies, ovarian wedge resection surgery removes a wedge section of the ovary, and the remaining edges are sewn together. The medical team of doctors

Stein and Leventhal was reported to have performed this type of surgery back in 1935, when PCOS was first diagnosed (and therefore referred to as Stein-Leventhal syndrome). Normal menstruation and even pregnancy was established in their patients receiving this surgery, making it the top surgical treatment for PCOS for several decades. Side effects of wedge resection, as with any surgery, can be scar tissue on the ovary that can ultimately cause infertility.

The success rates surrounding these procedures are often wide-ranging, and the studies and reports of their use can have differing results as well. If your doctor recommends one of these surgical procedures, do your research, ask to talk with women on whom the doctor has performed the procedure, and check PCOS chat sites and support groups for other women, outside your doctor's practice, who have gone this route. Then you will be making an informed decision for yourself.

Is Infertility a Sure Thing for Women with PCOS?

The short answer to this question is a resounding no! Many women with PCOS get pregnant, and many get pregnant without intervention, treatment, or even a diagnosis, for that matter. That's the thing about PCOS—nothing is "normal," and every woman who has the syndrome experiences a very unique condition.

However, despite the fact that almost everything has exceptions, women whose PCOS is causing anovulation—that is, no egg is being released—are, short of divine intervention, certainly going to experience infertility. Without an egg, there is no pregnancy. When the syndrome exhibits itself in other ways, infertility may not be an issue at all.

Three Steps to Pregnancy

There are three basic approaches for help, if you have difficulty getting pregnant. Your medical team—OB/GYN, primary care physician, reproductive endocrinologist—may want to try some or all. Typically, you would start with the least invasive and proceed to the more aggressive treatments. The three basic approaches are:

1. *Drug therapies:* As outlined in Chapter Five, "Medical Treatment for PCOS: Drugs and Surgical Options," there are many drugs that help women with PCOS. They range from hormone regulating agents to drugs to regulate your cycle, to plain old fertility drugs. Your reproductive endocrinologist should go through them all with you. If he or she doesn't, make sure to ask. This is where women who spend time doing research have made significant advances—by knowing what is out there and what to ask the doctor about specifically.

2. *Surgery:* Surgical options are largely for helping to alleviate PCOS symptoms that may be creating pregnancy problems. These options include the already mentioned "laparoscopic ovarian drilling" and ovarian wedge resection. Most of these surgeries are to restore function to the ovary and to trigger cycling and ovulation. Surgical interventions are usually only considered after less invasive procedures, such as drug therapies, have been tried and failed.

3. *Assisted pregnancy:* A key to getting pregnant may be the same assisted pregnancy techniques used by women who don't have PCOS but experience infertility for other reasons. In vitro fertilization, embryo transfer, and intrauterine insemination are all considered options for women with PCOS.

The Road to Pregnancy

You will work with your medical team—your OB/GYN, your endocrinologist, and other specialists—in creating a plan to get you on track toward pregnancy. There are many stages along that road. They include:

1. *Regulating your menstrual cycles:* If you do not menstruate at all or your cycles are irregular, you will work first on regulating them. We will discuss later in this chapter the various ways of doing that, but regular cycles are key to fertility.

2. *Ovulation:* You may get your menstrual cycles on track but find you are not actually ovulating—despite the fact that you experience cyclical bleeding, no egg is actually descending from the ovary. The reasons for this are myriad, but anovulation means no pregnancy will occur. You will want to work with your doctor to determine whether or not you are ovulating.

3. *Regulating your hormones:* Several different hormones are the keys to fertility. If your menstrual cycle has been regulated, chances are your hormones are normalizing as well, since they also have a major impact on your cycle. Getting insulin and, as a result, androgens under check is a major goal for women with PCOS, whether they are attempting to get pregnant or not.

Let's talk about how these three things can occur.

Regulating Menstrual Cycles

For women who are overweight, sometimes even a slight weight loss can stimulate a menstrual cycle. This may not be enough to sustain cycles, but modest weight loss for very overweight women can sometimes have a dramatic impact on cycling.

Menstruation can be induced with drugs. Sometimes the endometrial lining needs to thicken further to actually need to be shed; often cyclic estrogen and progesterone treatments can help tell the endometrial lining to thicken and shed, thus bringing on menses.

Even if you are not trying to get pregnant, the goal of regular menstrual cycles and, therefore, shedding of the endometrium is important, since retention of the lining is implicated in endometrial cancer.

Ovulation

If you have never had regular periods, regulating your cycle is the first step in getting to ovulation. However, as mentioned previously, you can be having menstrual cycles without ovulation occurring.

In order to determine whether or not your ovaries produce an egg during your cycle, you can purchase a simple "ovulation predictor kit"—a test designed to help you home in on the actual time frame of ovulation, the optimum time to try to conceive—although some of these kits even say on the package that they are unreliable for women with PCOS.

For ovulation to occur, there must be a surge of luteinizing hormone (LH) present. Ovulation predictor kits test for this elevated LH level in urine, which is indicated by the changing color on the test strip.

Nothing is infallible, and test kits can give false positives. Two possible reasons are that the LH level is heightened, but not enough to stimulate ovulation. Secondly, you always need to consider any medications you may be taking, especially ones that are intended to have an effect on hormones.

Regulating Your Hormones

The first step for hormone regulation is to be conscious of your diet and of good nutrition. (Is there an echo in here?) Diet and nutrition are simply the most effective way to begin controlling hormones. However, these two things alone are probably not going to be enough if you have PCOS with severe symptoms and difficulty getting pregnant. You could also try some of the complementary therapies discussed in Chapter Nine of this book, but there is limited research available to document their degree of efficacy.

The next best way to regulate hormones is probably drug therapy. Specifics are discussed in Chapter Five, but there are many drugs that are used to get hormones under control. Remember, when you have PCOS, trying to get pregnant does not mean exclusively regulating estrogen. Your treatment needs to go deeper than that, to the level of insulin regulation, which will ultimately work toward controlling estrogen and progesterone as well as androgens. Your reproductive endocrinologist will walk you through the hormonal maze.

Miscarriage

The jury is still out on the prevalence of miscarriage in women with PCOS. Early studies suggest that PCOS is associated with a higher incidence of miscarriage, but no real reason has been determined. When you become pregnant, probably the best thing you can do is be diligent about seeing your doctor, report anything that seems unusual, eat well, pace yourself but still get good exercise, and do all of the things that should be done by any pregnant woman who is devoted to taking care of herself and her unborn child. If a miscarriage happens, it's important not to blame yourself. If you did everything your doctor prescribed—such as getting complete bed rest—there is nothing you could have done to prevent a miscarriage. Repeat miscarriages can be especially trying; however, keep in mind that even after more than one miscarriage, you still have very good odds of carrying a child to term.

Some Natural Approaches

There are some things to do to help with pregnancy, some of which are just plain common sense and good for all women (and men!), some of which are specific to women with PCOS.

Diet: As mentioned, get your diet and nutrition on track. Good nutrition is the key to everything in your body.

Rid yourself of unhealthful habits: Avoid cigarette smoking, alcohol consumption, and caffeine when you are trying to get pregnant (and when you are pregnant). You simply don't need anything helping to make pregnancy more difficult. Your body needs to be at its optimum health.

Supplements: There are several vitamins, minerals, and herbs that are especially important for women with PCOS.

Stress reduction: PCOS symptoms and infertility have a way of raising your stress level. Mental stress triggers a series of changes in your body that further worsen PCOS symptoms and infertility. Stress creates its own vicious cycle of abnormal physiology—a storm that will rain all over your efforts to get pregnant. In fact, research has documented that the use of stress-reduction techniques can actually improve fertility in couples enrolled in infertility programs. The next chapter highlights several complementary/alternative therapies helpful in calming stress and improving your chances of pregnancy.

Patience and Persistence

Many of the personal stories found at the end of each chapter in this book are of women with PCOS who have become pregnant and are the proud moms of children. Many of them at one stage or another in their attempts to become pregnant were certain that it would never happen—and then, voila! The right combination of health care, medication, timing, and sometimes surgical intervention was what it took for the pregnancy test to come out positive.

Patience is hard, persistence is the key. Don't stress yourself and your partner so much that your attempt to start a family becomes a negative health factor and a negative influence on your relationship. Start early to tackle the symptoms that PCOS has brought your way—well before you seriously begin a plan to attempt pregnancy.

Don't let the stresses of regulating symptoms add on to the stresses of trying to become pregnant. And be comforted by the fact that, as many of the women in this book show, having PCOS and having a child are not mutually exclusive. A woman with PCOS can get pregnant, and quite likely it will happen to you!

A PERSONAL STORY

Mary

Mary has always felt as if her body had a mind of its own, not falling into any category described as "normal." So when the symptoms of PCOS started to arise, she simply ignored them as normal for her.

When she and her doctor did discuss some symptoms that suggested endometriosis—lack of periods, discomfort during intercourse—they decided to check out her ovaries. They found the classic cysts of PCOS. "My ovaries were completely covered," Mary says. She'd never had blood work, but her PCOS diagnosis was in hand.

However, Mary already had a son. Her doctor described his birth as a miracle, given her symptoms, and told her that she could not expect to be able to conceive again. "Then I won't be having any more children," Mary said, "because I won't do fertility treatments—I don't want multiple babies!"

A month later she returned to the doctor for preoperative work for a laparoscopy to investigate for endometriosis and to remove some of the cysts on her ovaries. At that pre-op meeting, she told the doctor she had taken a pregnancy test that came out positive. No laparoscopy for her. She did another pregnancy test, and the doctor did an ultrasound, and in Mary's words, "Bam! Babies." Twins! The doctor, she said, seemed to enjoy relating to her that she was having a "bonus baby." Two miracles in one, no treatments necessary.

Despite her lack of problems conceiving, Mary continued to have PCOS symptoms such as weight gain, moodiness, facial hair growth, abdominal pain, and very irregular periods.

The weight gain is the thing that bothers her the most, but she is just too busy and has become too accustomed to the weight to do anything about it. She has tried medication to treat PCOS symptoms, but finds that her body doesn't respond well to most drugs, so she chooses to deal with the PCOS symptoms rather than the medications' side effects.

Mary already eats a balanced, healthy diet of little red meat, lots of fruits and vegetables, and almost no junk food. She did some long-distance walking until the twin girls arrived; without sitters, she hasn't been able to get to a fitness center.

At this point in her life, Mary chooses to have her health take a backseat to the major responsibility in her life of parenting her three miracle babies! But she hasn't given up completely in her quest to get the answers she seeks, and she knows that someday it will become a priority for her.

CHAPTER NINE ∾

Alternative Approaches for Managing PCOS

For women with PCOS, everyday life is full of challenges. Happily, there are some useful natural strategies to improve the quality of your day-to-day life. Through alternative approaches and treatments, many women have found at least some relief from the frustrating symptoms that accompany PCOS. You, too, may be able to diminish symptoms, address some of the underlying causes, and improve overall health by taking advantage of natural approaches.

Simply taking an active role in exploring and using holistic approaches to health can help give life with PCOS a positive boost, too. To help you begin your exploration of a range of healing possibilities, this chapter will introduce you to several options that women have used to reduce the symptoms and stresses—physical and emotional—of PCOS, including acupuncture and other energy therapies, supplements, and herbal strategies.

Before You Begin
The Effects Take Time and Are Different for Everyone
Remember that not every approach, whether medical or alternative, provides the same benefits for everyone, so don't be discouraged if your results from one approach aren't as dramatic as you might hope. Visit the natural treatments chat list at the PCOA Web site at www.pcosupport.org to see what other women are doing to lessen the frustrations of PCOS. Work with your physician, network with other women, keep your hopes up, and try, try again.

Definition
First, it's important to define the two main words you will see when speaking of herbs, energy therapies, and other natural approaches: "alternative" and "complementary." In 2002, the Medical Subject Headings (MeSH) Section staff of the National Library of Medicine classified alternative medicine under the term "complementary therapies." These are defined as therapeutic practices that are not currently integrated into conventional Western medical practice. Therapies are termed "complementary" when used in addition to conventional treatments and "alternative" when used instead of conventional treatment. CAM (complementary and alternative medicine) is a broader, more general term that is widely used to refer to all "unconventional" therapies.

Sorting Through the Many Options
There are well over 300 CAM therapies, and it is very confusing to try to understand what's available and when it's appropriate to use which therapies. Some CAM therapies (such as acupuncture) have a fair amount of research behind them and a long track record of successful use. Other CAM therapies are supported by little or no research and have a negligible (or spotted) track record. There is so much marketing hyperbole that it often is hard to tell what's real and what's not.

One way to begin to make sense of it all is to group the many therapies into categories based on how we think they work. For instance the use of dietary measures, supplements, herbs, or vitamins has an impact on the biochemistry of your body—so we could call these "biochemical" therapies. Different massage techniques, chiropractic manipulation, and osteopathic manipulative therapy all affect the anatomic structures of the body. As it turns out, your stress hormones (adrenaline and cortisol) go down after a therapeutic massage, so there are also biochemical consequences, but the primary mechanism of action of massage and different manipulative techniques is work on the anatomic structures—therefore we could call these "structural" therapies. Exercise classes, tai chi, yoga, and other forms of dynamic activity could be classified as "movement" therapies. Avoidance of exposure to irritating or harmful influences in your environment (pesticides, hormones, pollutants, and so on) can be thought of as "environment-based" or "environmental" therapies. Stress-reducing techniques (whether you're talking about prayer, guided imagery, laughter/humor therapy, music therapy, counseling, or others) all work through the power of the mind to change your perception and response patterns. When your perceptions and responses change for the better, your body physiology follows with a decrease in the same stress hormones affected by massage. As a group we can consider these to be "mind-body" therapies. Finally, there are a number of therapies that seem to alter the balance or flow of charge—electromagnetic activity or energy flow in the body. Examples of these "energy" therapies include the use of acupuncture (which is a part of traditional Chinese medicine, or TCM), ayurveda (an ancient system of healing from India), therapeutic touch, Reiki, biomagnetics, and others. Interestingly, tai chi (which is a part of TCM) and yoga (which is a part of the ayurvedic system of healing) can also be considered energy therapies, since they are designed to achieve a balance and flow of energy through movement and can even be thought of as mind-body therapies because of their stress-reducing effects.

No classification system is perfect, but these six broad categories can be used to better understand what therapeutic options are available:

- Biochemical therapies
- Structural therapies
- Movement therapies
- Environmental therapies
- Mind-Body therapies
- Energy therapies

For the rest of this chapter, we will walk through the different categories and share examples of a number of specific therapies that may be helpful for women with PCOS.

Biochemical Therapies

Aside from the importance of diet, discussed in Chapter Six, there is an important role for nutritional supplements such as inositol, chromium, B complex, fenugreek, gymnema sylvestre, cinnamon, and FOS to decrease insulin requirements and improve insulin sensitivity. A number of other supplements may also be helpful depending of your specific symptoms.

Inositol

A specific form of inositol (d-chiroinositol) has been shown to decrease insulin resistance and improve symptoms in women with PCOS. D-chiroinositol seems to act as a messenger for insulin that transmits the message to the cell after insulin attaches to the receptors on the surface of the cell. The dose of d-chiroinositol used in the PCOS research was 1,200 milligrams per day.

However, you can't just go out to the health food store and buy this as a supplement. There are a few over-the-counter products that contain small amounts of d-chiroinositol as part of a multi-ingredient blend. Unfortunately these are body-building products used by weightlifters and are not exactly what you are looking for. The good news is that d-chiroinositol is not the only form of inositol that acts as an insulin messenger. Myoinositol seems to function in the same way, and this is the ingredient in the inositol supplements that are readily available at the health food store. An inositol dose of 750 to 1,000 milligrams twice daily is probably reasonable. You can also increase your inositol consumption substantially by consuming more beans. Beans have the double benefit of being a healthy, low glycemic-index food and a rich source of inositol. Another concentrated source of inositol is soy lecithin. Taking a couple of tablespoons of soy lecithin granules daily is a great way to get more inositol.

Chromium

Chromium appears to play a crucial role in the function of insulin. Research has documented that the use of chromium piccolinate or chromium polynicotinate can improve blood-sugar control with doses up to 1,000 micrograms used per day in diabetic patients. More is not better, and I would definitely not recommend taking higher doses. Taking 200 micrograms of one of these chromium products two to three times daily with meals should be plenty.

B-Complex Vitamins

Niacinamide is a form of vitamin B3 that can increase insulin sensitivity. Niacin, on the other hand, if taken in high doses (1,000 milligrams per day or more), could worsen insulin sensitivity. Biotin is another B vitamin that appears to improve insulin sensitivity. A high-dose multivitamin usually will contain extra amounts of the B vitamins that can help insulin work better in your body. Another option is to take a separate B-50 or B-100 complex daily. When shopping for B-complex, look for one that has more niacinamide than niacin.

Fenugreek

Fenugreek is an herb that interferes with the absorption and digestion of sugars. In this sense it is somewhat like the insulin-sparing prescription medicines—acarbose and miglitol. Fenugreek tends to be bitter, but if you use the defatted fenugreek powder (25-50 grams twice daily with meals), it is more tolerable. While you can take fenugreek in capsule form to avoid the bitter taste, that would be an awful lot of capsules to gag down. By the way, don't take fenugreek during pregnancy, as it stimulates lactation and uterine contractions.

Gymnema Sylvestre

Gymnema sylvestre is an herb that comes to us from the ayurvedic tradition of healing. It seems to improve insulin sensitivity, and like fenugreek, can also interfere with sugar absorption. In contrast to fenugreek, the doses used for gymnema are only 400-500 mg daily—much easier to handle than 50-100 grams per day!

Cinnamon

In preliminary findings, cinnamon helped fat cells recognize and respond to insulin. In studies conducted by the Beltsville, Maryland, Human Nutrition Center, a branch of the Department of Agriculture (USDA), the spice appeared to increase glucose metabolism by about twenty times. It contains a phytochemical called methylhydroxychalcone polymer (MHCP), which improves cellular glucose utilization and increases the sensitivity of insulin receptors. Try adding a teaspoon a day to cereal or other foods.

Fructo-oligosaccharide (FOS)

FOS, 1 gram daily, can normalize blood sugar levels in cases of insulin resistance, as well as lower elevated cholesterol levels. This complex sugar is not broken down by digestive juices as other sugars are. In the intestine, it nourishes the "good" bacteria that aid digestion, enhance immune function, maintain correct acidity levels in the gastrointestinal tract, and control the growth of fungi and "bad" bacteria that can cause yeast infections and gastric disorders.

Other Useful Supplements
Black Cohosh (cimcifuga racemosa)
Widely used by American Indians and colonial Americans for the relief of menstrual cramps and menopausal symptoms, black cohosh may also restore suppressed menstruation. The herb has substances that bind to estrogen receptors and lower LH (a hormone that is elevated in menopause). An added benefit is that black cohosh can also lower blood pressure slightly. The majority of the research has been done with Remifemin, a brand of black cohosh produced originally in Germany according to stringent quality-control measures. In the United States we still haven't caught up with Germany in terms of regulating and enforcing quality-control standards for herbs and supplements. Standardization and quality control are good because they usually lead to more predictable results and a better safety margin. Remifemin is standardized to have 1 mg of 27-deoxyacteine, one of the main active ingredients, per tablet. A typical dose is one or two tablets twice daily.

Chasteberries (vitex agnus castus)
In two surveys of over 1,500 women in German gynecological practices, chasteberry extract was graded as good or very good in treating the symptoms of PMS. The extract is particularly useful in cases of corpus luteum insufficiency, common in PCOS cases, because it has profound effects on the hypothalmus (see Chapter Two) and pituitary function. It can normalize the secretion of hormones, reduce the secretion of prolactin, and lower the estrogen-progesterone ratio. It can take three months to lower prolactin levels, so be patient. Use 175-225 mg a day in capsule form or 2 ml a day of liquid.

Natural Progesterone Cream

Although applied topically to the skin rather than taken internally, natural progesterone creams allow you to absorb progesterone that is identical to the natural hormone produced in your body. Progesterone plays a major role in regulating menstruation. Progesterone can decrease the risk of endometrial cancer—this is particularly relevant in women who have PCOS. Many women with PCOS have had success using progesterone cream to stimulate regular periods. A typical dose is ¼ to ½ teaspoon of natural progesterone cream applied twice daily.

5-Hydroxytryptophan (5-HTP)

Depression is common in women with PCOS. 5-HTP, which is converted to serotonin in your body, has been shown to be effective for mild to moderate depression. 5-HTP has also been demonstrated to help control appetite during weight-loss programs. A typical dose of 5-HTP would be 50-100 milligrams, on an empty stomach, up to twice daily. 5-HTP should generally not be combined with prescription antidepressant medicines because of the potential for dangerous interactions.

S-Adenosylmethionine (SAMe)

SAMe is another supplement with documented efficacy in mild to moderate depression. Doses of SAMe are usually in the range of 400-800 mg twice a day. It's not uncommon to pay $1.00 per 200-mg pill of SAMe, so you can see that this could be a pretty pricey supplement in the recommended doses. Unlike 5-HTP, SAMe is OK to use along with prescription antidepressants.

St. John's Wort

St. John's Wort has been studied extensively and shown to be of benefit for patients with mild to moderate depression. The dose found effective in the studies has been 300 mg three times daily of a product standardized to 0.3 percent hypericin. The other side of St. John's

Wort, though, is that it revs up your liver metabolism and lowers the blood levels of many prescription drugs you might be taking. The result is that St. John's Wort ends up decreasing the effectiveness of prescription drugs by speeding their elimination from your body. So while St. John's Wort may be beneficial, it should not be used with most prescription medicines.

Supplements to Avoid

As already mentioned earlier in this chapter, high doses of niacin should be avoided, as this can worsen insulin sensitivity. As discussed in the diet chapter, weight-loss products containing ephedra (ma huang) are too unpredictable and are best avoided because of safety concerns. Another popular supplement to be careful with is glucosamine sulfate. The amount of actual glucose in glucosamine sulfate is not enough to have a significant impact on glucose. However, by a mechanism that is not entirely understood, glucosamine has been shown to increase insulin resistance.

What to Look for on the Bottle

Because of the lax regulatory policies in the United States for establishing herb and supplement quality control, there is huge variability in the quality of products on the market. Therefore, you need to know what to look for, to be able to distinguish the winners from the duds. As highlighted in the section on black cohosh, standardization is a good thing. The manufacturer should state on the label how many milligrams there are of each ingredient and, when possible, indicate the percentages of active ingredients. From a quality control perspective, the bottle should mention a batch number, lot number, and expiration date. From a customer service perspective, there should be a company address, phone number, and return policy on the bottle. It would be nice if there were research available using the specific product you are considering, instead of research on a similar product. Perhaps one of the most important things to look for is an indication of independent laboratory verification of the contents. Having an unbiased third party (who has no vested interest in selling you products) verify that the bottle actually contains what's on the label (and does not contain adulterants or contaminants not listed on the label) is extremely valuable. ConsumerLab (www.consumerlab.com) and USP, the United States Pharmocopeia (www.usp.org), are a couple of organizations that have established laboratory verification programs to help consumers identify more reputable and reliable brands of herbs and supplements.

A Word to the Wise

Whatever herbs or supplements you are considering taking, be sure to tell your doctor. There can sometimes be serious drug-herb-supplement interactions, particularly when the right hand doesn't know what the left hand is doing. Prescription medicines are also biochemical interventions, and their effects can be dangerously enhanced or diminished when combined with some herbs or supplements. Drugs that have a "narrow therapeutic window" (such as blood thinners like warfarin or heart medicines like digoxin) are particularly vulnerable to bad interactions. But even if you're not on one of these medicines, be sure to talk to your doctor about any herbs or supplements you are using.

Structural Therapies

While massage or manipulative therapies do not directly treat PCOS, having a massage periodically is a healthy thing to do. Not only does a therapeutic massage make you feel relaxed and improve circulation and range of motion, but the documented decreases in blood cortisol and adrenaline levels are good for you. These two stress hormones can increase glucose levels and insulin resistance.

Movement Therapies

In Chapter Seven we discussed the importance of exercise and mentioned how yoga, a specific type of movement therapy, can be beneficial. Here we will highlight in more detail the role yoga can play.

Yoga: Moving the Body and Calming the Mind

Yoga is a gentle form of movement that, according to the ayurvedic healing tradition, helps balance the flow of energy (called "prana" by ayurvedic practitioners) in the body. Diaphragmatic breathing techniques are an integral part of yoga practice. People under stress commonly assume a shallow chest-breathing pattern that actually tends to worsen anxiety and tension. Deep diaphragmatic breathing can be both physically invigorating and mentally calming. Yoga has been practiced for thousands of years in India and is now used widely throughout the world to increase suppleness and vitality and relieve stress.

The most popular form of yoga in the West is hatha yoga, "hatha" meaning balance. Asanas, the series of body postures used to develop flexibility and controlled relaxation, are performed slowly and deliberately to benefit both mind and body. Controlled breathing regulates prana in the body.

Beginners will benefit from joining a class run by a qualified teacher, who can correct postures and help improve relaxation techniques. Correct body position during the asanas is vital to their effectiveness. Most classes last forty to ninety minutes and begin with a gentle warm-up.

If you practice alone, progress gradually through the postures. Asanas should never cause severe pain, though some aches in muscles that haven't been used or stretched for a while can be expected. Some people have had good success using yoga videos as teachers. Work near a mirror so you can confirm that your postures and alignment are correct. Practice for twenty to thirty minutes a day to increase energy and stamina, tone muscles, improve digestion, enhance concentration, and reduce stress. Be sure to allow two to three hours after a meal before you practice.

Environmental Therapies

There are a number of studies suggesting that exposure to "xenoestrogens" (estrogen-like chemicals in the environment), pesticides, and hormones could disrupt hormonal function. While there is some debate and controversy surrounding these theories, you can't go wrong by eating more organic foods and drinking filtered water. Perhaps even more controversial is the role that chronic exposure to low-level electromagnetic fields may have in illness. Although it is possible to find research supporting almost any viewpoint, it is fascinating that laboratory animals exposed chronically to low levels of electromagnetic fields tend to have higher cortisol levels—a classic physiologic stress response that is associated with more insulin resistance. This doesn't mean that you have to throw away all your appliances and go live in a cave. On the other hand, you may want to pull the plug on your electric blanket or waterbed at night, and not sit directly under fluorescent lights all day.

Mind-Body Therapies

Any therapy that lowers stress levels is a plus for women with PCOS. Obviously, stress-lowering therapies can be a good thing for anyone, but they are even more beneficial in the face of insulin resistance. The way the body responds when the mind perceives stress is to pump out more cortisol and adrenalin, which in turn raises glucose levels and worsens insulin resistance.

Counseling

Counseling can often help you identify perceptions and dysfunctional coping strategies that can be a self-imposed source of stress. Perceptions and coping strategies are both within your control, and learning to change these and use them to your advantage instead of letting them work against you can be enormously liberating. Sometimes, as the saying goes, we are our own worst enemies. A good counselor can help you be better to yourself and reduce your stress levels considerably.

The H-P-A Axis

The H-P-A axis is short for hypothalamic-pituitary-adrenal axis. Repeat after me three times quickly: "hypothalamic-pituitary-adrenal axis"! Well on second thought, skip the repeating and let's stick with H-P-A axis. What this really means is that scientists have identified how our thoughts and emotions can be translated by our bodies into dramatic physiologic consequences. The hypothalamus, a master regulatory center in the brain, receives input from the hippocampus and other parts of the brain associated with strong feelings and emotions. These inputs affect the electrical and chemical signals from the hypothalamus to the pituitary, a pea-sized gland located at the base of the brain. Don't let the pea-size fool you, because the pituitary gland in turn produces hormones that are released into your bloodstream to control all the endocrine glands in your body (thyroid, ovaries, adrenals, etc.). When the hippocampus sends your hypothalamus a "stress signal," the hypothalamus responds by sending CRH (corticotrophin-releasing hormone) to the pituitary gland. The pituitary then releases ACTH (adrenocorticotropic hormone) into the bloodstream. When the adrenal glands get bathed in ACTH, they squeeze out cortisol and adrenalin to prepare your body for "fight or flight."

As a result, your blood pressure and heart rate go up, as do your glucose and insulin resistance. Blood gets shifted away from your skin and digestive tract to the muscles, equipping you to do battle or flee. Your pupils dilate to heighten your perception, and your blood begins to clot more easily, just in case you are injured.

This entire cascade of events and much more is triggered in just seconds by a simple stressful thought or emotion that was transmitted and translated to your body as "get ready for the worst possible scenario." This can be a marvelous and life-saving thing if you are about to be run over by a bus or attacked by a thug, but it is not so great if triggered by watching the news, reading the newspaper, driving to work, or disagreeing with a coworker, friend, or spouse. The H-P-A axis does all of this faithfully on autopilot, without any effort or conscious thought required from us. But what if the autopilot is set to send out the "worst possible scenario" alarm at all times for the slightest disturbance? Over time this overly sensitive alarm takes its toll on your body and increases the risk of a number of diseases, both chronic (such as PCOS, diabetes, hypertension, and heart disease) and acute (such as a heart attack or stroke). Fortunately, there are a number of approaches that can be used to reset an overly sensitive H-P-A autopilot. Prayer, guided imagery, meditation, biofeedback, laughter/humor therapy, journal keeping, and music therapy are all excellent examples of approaches that have been used successfully to tone down an overly sensitive H-P-A autopilot. Find out which approaches you feel most comfortable using, and then incorporate them into your daily routine. I'm not suggesting an unrealistic goal of no stress in your life. The goal is to take active steps to better manage stress so as not to let it make you sick (or worse).

Energy Therapies

There are many different interventions in this category, but I think acupuncture serves as the best example or prototype to convey how these therapies can greatly contribute to improving the health of women with PCOS.

Acupuncture Basics

Before communication was reopened with China thirty years ago, acupuncture was extremely rare in the Western world. Today, acupuncture is a widely accepted and widely practiced medical modality. Its use extends into mainstream medicine in the United States and throughout the world.

The traditional Chinese medicine (TCM) health system that includes acupuncture, as well as herbs, acupressure, exercise, and diet, is based in part on the concept of a universal life energy known as qi (pronounced "chi"). Qi includes the spiritual, emotional, mental, and physical aspects of life. A person's health is said to be influenced by the flow of qi; the even circulation of qi around the body is thought to be essential for good health.

Qi is comprised of two elements, yin and yang, which are opposite forces that work together when balanced. Qi travels throughout the body along meridians—pathways located just below the surface of the skin. Energy constantly flows up and down these pathways. When meridians become obstructed, deficient, excessive, or uneven, yin and yang are said to be out of balance, which can cause illness. Acupuncture's goal is to restore balance and, as a result, good health.

To skeptical, Western-trained researchers, qi, yin, yang, and universal life energy are concepts that are viewed as foreign, and often, nonsensical. The Western mindset is to measure and quantify whenever possible. As it turns out, the acupuncture meridians and acupuncture points (hundreds of points that lie directly over the meridians and have been called "reactive electropermeable points" by some researchers) can be reproducibly detected as low-resistance electrical pathways. Insertion of an acupuncture needle or application of pressure (acupressure) at the acupoints induces electrical changes in the tissues, and the flow of minute electrical currents along the low-resistance pathways (paths of least resistance). Researchers have also shown that pathology (whether it be a tumor, a cut, a fracture, a muscle spasm, or a headache) can be associated with abnormal electrical activity, and that correction of the abnormal electrical activity can speed or facilitate the healing process. The concept of energy and physiology being intimately linked therefore has a solid foundation. Despite the persuasive evidence, this way of understanding body function has not been widely accepted in the West. There is such a large amount of research supporting its effectiveness that there is little debate as to whether or not acupuncture works. The debate is, rather, about how acupuncture works. A number of alternate theories have been proposed by skeptics unwilling to accept the energy-based explanation. Some attribute all of the effects of acupuncture to the release of pain-relieving endorphins, since endorphin blockers neutralize the pain-relieving effect of acupuncture. Others invoke "gating" of nerve signals along complex neurologic circuits to explain how acupuncture works. Since there is evidence supporting all these positions and nothing to suggest that these mechanisms are in any way mutually exclusive, the right answer is probably: e.) all of the above.

A Typical Visit

On your first visit to a licensed acupuncturist, you will be asked questions about your condition and lifestyle as part of the assessment process, which is based on the arts of asking, observing, listening, and touching—the Four examinations central to TCM. On each wrist, there are six meridian pulses that your acupuncturist will check. She may also check your tongue for imbalances in yin and yang (you may want to avoid any food or drink that will color your tongue before your visit). After the assessment process, an energy diagnosis is established. Rather than a familiar diagnosis such as "PCOS with infertility, acne, and obesity," you might hear something like "Qi stagnation of the liver and yin deficiency of the kidney." The goal of treatment is to correct the energy imbalance, and not specifically to treat PCOS with infertility and the rest. Twenty different women with PCOS may have twenty different energy diagnoses, and the treatment recommendations for each one will be different. You will discuss treatment options, followed perhaps by advice on lifestyle and diet. In some cases, Chinese herbal medicine may be recommended.

Before treatment, you'll remove clothing that covers the acupoints to be treated, typically located on the back, abdomen, shoulders, face, head, hands, and feet. Treatment usually involves a combination of acupoints. Needles are inserted quickly and painlessly and may be left in place for a few seconds or as much as an hour. The practitioner may gently twist the needle to regulate qi flow. When the session is over, the needles are withdrawn and leave no trace on your skin.

Another acupoint stimulation option is acupressure. This is basically acupuncture without needles. Stimulation of the acupuncture points is performed with the fingers or an instrument with a hard, ball-shaped head. You may even stimulate points yourself. Your acupuncturist may give you suggestions for points to focus on between visits.

Visit www.acupuncture.com to learn about how to locate a licensed practitioner in the states that license the profession. Here's an acupuncture testimonial from a PCOS chat site:

"Acupuncture takes a while to work but let me tell you it is worth it. I am almost afraid to get too excited, like this is a fluke or something...but I believe in my heart that it isn't. Believe me, I've been right up there with the most discouraged people on this list in the past. If you aren't having results, stick with it! I've had doctors tell me that my only hope was meds. A lot of my symptoms have been improved by the acupuncture and other mind-body approaches."

Energy Exercises
Another fundamental component of TCM energy work is exercise. To facilitate health through the improved flow of qi, people around the world follow such gentle exercise practices as qi gong and tai chi on a

regular basis. Both are considered noncombative martial arts that use breathing techniques and sequences of slow, graceful movements to supple and strengthen the body, promote self-healing, and calm the mind and spirit. You may find that you feel more energetic and strong after regular practice.

Other Energy Therapies

The concept of the flow of energy within and around the body lies at the heart of many other therapies, including shiatsu, magnetic therapy, therapeutic touch, and Reiki, to name a few. The amount of research and experience with acupuncture is much greater than what is typically available with other energy therapies. But this doesn't mean people don't do well with these other techniques. Reiki, for instance, is a gentle hands-on energy technique that has very little research to support it, compared to acupuncture. The training process for Reiki practitioners is also not as standardized or rigorous as that for acupuncture and other forms of TCM. Despite the limited research and greater variability in practitioner skills, however, many patients have had great responses to Reiki, such as this one: *"I have a friend who is a Reiki healer and although I don't have any proof that the sessions help with PCOS, they certainly leave me feeling relaxed and stress free! I try to go and see her at least once a month, because I feel so great after each session, and I look on it in the same way as having a facial!"*

Where Do You Begin?

Awareness is power. It's been said in this book before, but it bears repeating: There may be a silver lining within the cloud of a PCOS diagnosis. While you won't have the luxury of taking your good health for granted, becoming your own health advocate during the PCOS journey may ultimately open the door to a more vibrant and vigorous life. The key is awareness that there are options available.

The power of natural remedies to improve the quality of life after a PCOS diagnosis relies on identifying one or more combinations of strategies and/or remedies to help your body rally. So where do you start? Use the information in this chapter to begin your exploration of complementary/alternative coping tactics. Consult your current health care provider about natural options. Find a PCOS support group and ask lots of questions. The experiences of other women dealing naturally with PCOS may be very useful for identifying beneficial strategies, but keep in mind that PCOS affects each woman a bit differently, and as the saying goes, your results may vary. Whatever therapies you decide to use, be sure to monitor the effectiveness of what you're doing. Keep a detailed symptom diary and include weights, menstrual cycles, and whatever else is relevant. Determine in advance how long you are willing to try a therapy before concluding that it's not doing what you want and it's time to move on to something else. Don't keep doing more of the same if it's not working for you. If less aggressive approaches aren't enough, then it may be time to step up to more aggressive strategies to get the results you want.

Arm yourself with information about the wealth of possibilities, and get ready to meet the challenges of life with PCOS head-on. Use this chapter as a springboard for further education on natural remedies and alternative/complementary approaches, and work with a health care provider who can help guide you through the various options. It is important that your health care provider view you as a unique individual with physical, mental, and spiritual needs, not just as a disease with a person inconveniently attached. A health care provider with a holistic, patient-centered philosophy will strive to ensure that your care is comprehensive in scope and personalized by design. Any health care provider who does this will, of necessity, be collaborative in nature, because no one practitioner has mastery of all the competencies and skill sets to meet all the needs of someone with a complex condition like

PCOS. A team of practitioners is much better able to respond to your needs than any one practitioner. You are the captain of that team, but a knowledgeable health care provider with a balanced, integrative philosophy can be an invaluable co-captain who helps you get the most out of the team. Add some positive thinking, the tincture of time, and a little support. Your explorations of the rewarding world of complementary/alternative healing therapies may lead to better health than you thought possible.

A PERSONAL STORY

Lenke

Touring with a musical group in Europe in 1990, Lenke got the flu. After recovering, she was startled by a rapid gain in weight—thirty-five pounds in two months! Acne followed immediately after that, and hair-growth issues came on strong.

"I wondered, of course, if my body was reacting to the food," Lenke says. They were on the road a lot, and between that and new foods in new countries, it was a logical suspicion. She mentioned it to her parents, but didn't take it further than that at the moment.

"I came home at the holidays to surprise my parents with a visit," she said. When they opened the door, Lenke's own parents didn't recognize her. She had cut her hair, but she knew that wasn't the problem.

Lenke had been a reasonable size 10 for her overall body shape, but now her clothing size jumped to a 16. When she came home that summer, she went to a clinic. They did a CAT scan of her brain, took an ultrasound of her ovaries, and checked hormone levels. The ultrasound showed the classic cysts, and her hormone levels showed high testosterone. The PCOS/insulin connection hadn't yet been made, and so they didn't test her insulin levels.

Her doctor put her on the pill. Lenke resumed her travels for a year, but continued to find it hard to make her own food choices. She decided she needed to focus on her health, came home, and spent one year completely focused on diet and exercise. She dropped to her current size 6, and her doctors were shocked by what the weight loss and increased fitness did to her body, reworking her entire hormone levels and metabolism.

"I still had the symptoms but felt a lot better," she says. She went on the pill and spironolactone, and started to gain control of the emotional roller-coaster side of PCOS. The drug helped control the acne and hair-growth issues, although they didn't go completely away.

In June of 2000, Lenke went on metformin, and in four months, she became pregnant. She went off it a few weeks into her pregnancy, as is necessary, and she has never gone back to metformin because it made her feel sick.

"I am often referred to as a 'thin cyster' in PCOS circles," Lenke says, "but I wasn't always that way. I now carry two pictures of myself with me: one of me thin, and one of the not-thin me. People don't recognize that they are photos of the same person."

The weight-control and exercise part of PCOS management has been a very serious thing for Lenke. She said, "PCOS is not controlling my life; I don't let it. I look beyond it as best I can."

CHAPTER TEN ∾

Management and Prognosis

Excluding Other Diagnoses

The first step in proper management is establishing a clear diagnosis. While a history of weight gain, irregular/missed periods, infertility, acne, hirsutism, and alopecia is very suggestive of PCOS, there are other conditions that could produce many of the same symptoms. Because of this it is helpful to do a few tests—not so much to confirm a diagnosis of PCOS as to exclude other conditions.

A prolactin-producing pituitary tumor, thyroid disorders, and adrenal hyperplasia are all examples of medical conditions that might mimic PCOS. As obvious as it may seem, pregnancy is also an overlooked cause of weight gain and missed periods. Aside from a pregnancy test, it is reasonable to do blood tests for prolactin, cortisol (an adrenal hormone), DHEA-sulfate (an adrenal androgen), testosterone, TSH (thyroid-stimulating hormone), and free T3 (the last two are thyroid tests). With PCOS you would expect to find a negative pregnancy test, normal to mildly elevated prolactin, normal to moderately elevated DHEA-sulfate and testosterone, and normal thyroid tests. If the prolactin is more than mildly elevated, a pituitary tumor is likely. If the DHEA-sulfate and testosterone are dramatically elevated, the possibility of an adrenal tumor should be explored. The thyroid tests are generally normal in patients with PCOS, but it may be helpful to briefly discuss what this really means.

"Normal" Tests, Real Suffering

A significant number of patients who suffer with chronic complaints for years (and sometimes decades) are subjected to repeat diagnostic testing to no avail. In the absence of laboratory abnormalities to explain the symptoms, patients and physicians are frustrated in their attempts to determine a diagnosis. It is both easy and unfortunate for clinicians to be fooled into thinking that there is no serious illness because the lab tests are normal. If in fact there is pathology in the face of normal tests, we should reexamine, clarify, and perhaps even redefine what we mean by "normal."

What is Normal?

Laboratory testing of a healthy individual is subject to fluctuations based on a number of factors, including activity, age, diurnal hormone swings, environmental factors, and nutritional state. With enough data points for any individual, it is possible to statistically determine a range for a given laboratory parameter that encompasses 95 percent of values (the mean plus or minus two standard deviations). Values outside of this range are unlikely and increase suspicions of pathology or laboratory error. Values within the range are considered statistically expected ("normal"), and values outside of the range are considered statistically unexpected ("abnormal").

When performing laboratory testing on a population, researchers perform a similar statistical analysis to determine normal reference ranges for any given parameter. Variability within a population includes all of the intra-individual factors already mentioned, and it also includes significant inter-individual factors such as gender and genetics. Therefore it is axiomatic and mathematically provable that the expected range for a healthy population is by definition greater than the expected range for a particular healthy individual. Another way of stating this is that the physiologic "comfort zone" of an individual is always narrower than the physiologic comfort zone for a population.

Normal for a Population Is Not Necessarily Normal for an Individual

Since the range of statistically expected laboratory values for a given parameter is always greater for a population than an individual, it is possible for an individual to have a laboratory test that is clearly abnormal (unexpected) for her but that still falls within what is considered normal for a population. In other words, the domain of normal values for a population includes both normal and abnormal values for a given individual. Therefore when laboratory analysis of a symptomatic patient reveals a test result that is skewed in one direction (but still within the statistically normal range for a population), it is possible that the result is abnormal for that individual—particularly if the skew of the test is in the same direction as the symptom skew.

A simple illustration of this principle can be seen with thyroid testing. The most commonly used test to screen for thyroid disease is the test for thyroid-stimulating hormone. The normal reference range for TSH (depending on the specific laboratory, equipment, reagents, and testing methodology used) is generally 0.5 to 5.0. This tenfold range encompasses what is expected for a population. Because of the feedback loop between the thyroid gland and pituitary glands, a higher TSH is associated with lower thyroid function, and vice versa.

If a patient presents with the onset of fatigue, poor concentration, weight gain, cold intolerance, constipation, irregular periods, and hair loss, and her TSH reading is 4.5, both the symptom skew and laboratory skew are compatible with hypothyroidism (low thyroid function). If by chance the patient has previous laboratory testing on file that showed a TSH of 1.0 ten years ago, 2.5 five years ago, and 3.5 two years ago, this would add further credence to the idea that a TSH of 4.5 may in fact be abnormal for her.

In this situation it is reasonable to treat the patient with a low dose of thyroid medicine and monitor both the symptoms and subsequent TSH readings to validate (or invalidate) the clinical suspicion of hypothyroidism, and make appropriate adjustments as needed. The goal would be to shift the TSH reading from 4.5 to the 1-2 range. Unfortunately, the vast majority of patients described in this scenario are still told that their lab tests are normal and that they do not have hypothyroidism. These patients are victims of a statistical mirage, a mathematical misunderstanding that condemns them to visiting doctor after doctor for years, miserable, dysfunctional, and disillusioned.

Laboratory Tools, Clinical Judgment Rules
While the use of laboratory testing is a powerful aid in diagnosis and treatment, we must not forget that it is merely a tool and, like any tool, can be misused. The proper use of laboratory testing is as an adjunct to clinical judgment, not a replacement. The misguided misinterpretation of population normalcy as individual normalcy is an example of the improper use of laboratory testing. Astute clinical judgment trumps crudely wielded laboratory tools. Although suffering is generally considered subjective and laboratory tests are considered objective, the practice of medicine dare not sacrifice the reality of subjectivity on the illusory altar of objectivity.

Even though physicians are taught in medical training to "treat the patient, not the labs," it is something that doctors must be frequently reminded of. As a patient, one thing you can (and probably should) do to decrease the likelihood of falling into the "normal trap" is to always ask for a copy of your tests. Don't just take the doctor's word for it that everything is normal. If your test results are at one end of the normal range (the same end that coincides with the symptoms you are having), this may be worth pursuing further.

Fine-Tuning a Diagnosis of PCOS

FSH and LH, the two pituitary hormones that regulate ovarian function, are generally out of balance in patients with PCOS. The FSH is usually normal to slightly low, and the LH is often moderately high; the combination of these imbalances produces an LH/FSH ratio of greater than three to one. Monitoring worsening or improvement of the LH/FSH ratio can provide an indication of the degree of pituitary imbalance and the success of treatment strategies. A pelvic ultrasound can sometimes show a ring of small cysts around the periphery of the ovaries. The presence of this finding on ultrasound helps to confirm the diagnosis of PCOS, but the absence of this finding by no means excludes a diagnosis of PCOS. The presence of ovarian cysts on ultrasound does not correlate well with the degree of hormonal imbalance, so serial ultrasounds are not particularly helpful for making management decisions in patients with PCOS.

Many, but not all, women with PCOS (even the 25-50 percent who are not obese) have problems with insulin resistance and are at greater risk of type 2 diabetes (four times as likely). In light of this it is reasonable to check fasting glucose and insulin levels. If the fasting insulin reading is greater than 20 units/ml or the glucose/insulin ratio is less than 4.5, this confirms the presence of insulin resistance and compensatory hyperinsulinemia. Since 20-40 percent of women with PCOS have an abnormal glucose tolerance test, this test may also be warranted, even though it takes three hours to do and is inconvenient. Documenting the presence and degree of insulin resistance is important in guiding treatment decisions.

In addition to the insulin-related problems, individuals with PCOS are at increased risk for developing hypertension (2.5 times as likely) and heart disease. Monitoring kidney function tests (BUN and creatinine) and lipids (total cholesterol, LDL, HDL, and triglycerides) is appropriate as part of screening and management for these associated conditions.

Where to Begin?

After an adequate workup to establish and fine-tune a diagnosis has been done, treatment decisions are usually prioritized according to which symptoms are most bothersome (or most dangerous). Since PCOS can, for the most part, be considered a chronic condition with no immediate danger of losing life or limb, it is entirely logical and appropriate to start with interventions that are the least aggressive, least risky, least expensive, and most in your control. Monitoring the success of these interventions for a predetermined time frame will determine whether or not the use of more aggressive measures is called for.

The first steps always include diet and exercise, as discussed in previous chapters. A low glycemic-index diet will decrease insulin levels. However, a low glycemic-index diet should not be misinterpreted as an unbalanced high-protein, high-fat, no-carbohydrate diet. A well-balanced low glycemic-index diet includes plenty of fruits, vegetables, and whole grains that provide complex carbohydrates and a host of essential nutrients. It's also worth remembering that there are no benefits of a 10,000-calorie-per-day low glycemic-index diet. Excessive calories are a problem regardless of the source. In addition to a restricted-calorie, low glycemic-index diet, the use of certain supplements that enhance the effectiveness of insulin (such as inositol, chromium, B-complex vitamins, and/or cinnamon) or decrease the demand for insulin (herbs such as fenugreek or gymnema sylvestre) can be beneficial. The cinnamon, by the way, should ideally not be attached to a cinnamon bun!

Since stress and inadequate/irregular sleep are known to raise cortisol, sugar, and insulin levels, stress management and regular sleeping hours are critical. Regular exercise is certainly one effective way of lowering stress levels. Other effective tools to reduce stress include humor, diaphragmatic/yoga breathing techniques, prayer, journal keeping, meditation, aromatherapy, therapeutic massage, acupuncture, and counseling if needed.

Next Steps

If the initial self-help steps prove inadequate, then it's time to add prescription medicines. The chapter on drug and surgical treatments outlines what's available and how these treatments are used. If insulin resistance has been documented, the insulin sensitizers (such as Glucophage/metformin) and the insulin-sparing agents (such as Precose/Acarbose) would be a logical first recommendation, because they would help with all the symptoms of PCOS from hair loss to unwanted hair growth, to acne, to irregular periods, to infertility, to weight gain. With both metformin and Acarbose (as with most medicines), it is best to start at the lowest dose (500 mg daily for metformin and 25 mg daily for Acarbose) and work up to a maintenance dose to reduce the likelihood of side effects. Periodic monitoring of liver and kidney function tests with these medicines can also identify potential problems early and decrease the chance of untoward events due to medication use.

Last Steps

If the use of insulin sensitizers and insulin-sparing agents has not been effective enough to achieve the desired goals, then medicines and/or treatments can be chosen based on the particular symptoms and concerns of the individual patient. If infertility is the primary issue, then clomiphene might be used. If hirsutism and alopecia are most bothersome, then antiandrogens might be tried. If obesity is the main issue, weight-loss medications may be called for. The manifestations of PCOS are different for every affected woman, and the treatment approach should reflect this reality. There is no "one-size-fits-all" treatment regimen for patients with PCOS. However, the benefit of any medical or surgical treatment will be enhanced and maximized by the use of diet, exercise, appropriate supplements, stress reduction, and management of insulin resistance. Immediately jumping to the last steps without conscientiously going through the first and second steps of management is associated with poor outcomes and increased complications. This would be akin to aggressively treating asthma patients with high steroid doses, allergy shots, inhalers, and half a dozen other medications without first having them stop smoking.

Prognosis

There is persuasive evidence supporting a genetic basis (probably autosomal dominant) for PCOS. If this is true, the question that naturally arises is, "If PCOS is programmed into my genes, what's the point of trying to treat it? Won't any efforts just be an exercise in futility?" In fact, nothing could be further from the truth. While the propensity to develop insulin resistance (which in turn leads to the many symptoms of PCOS) may be genetically programmed, lifestyle measures and, if needed, medications can prevent or reverse insulin resistance and all of the associated problems.

To give a specific illustration, recent research using metformin in nonobese, nonovulating PCOS patients documented a 93 percent ovulation rate by the fifth and sixth months of the study, whereas none of the patients who received a placebo ovulated during the study. Perhaps the most interesting finding in this study is that, even though there was a very dramatic response to the insulin sensitizing effects of metformin, none of the patients had insulin resistance (as defined by the laboratory parameters mentioned earlier in this chapter). This suggests that, to some extent, all women with PCOS have an element of insulin resistance, even when the tests available are not sophisticated enough to be able to detect it. The historical success rates in treating infertility, acne, hirsutism, and obesity in patients with PCOS have been nowhere near 90 percent. The focus on treating insulin resistance has been relatively recent, and there has not yet been enough research to give accurate statistics to predict response rates for the different symptoms of PCOS using this new emphasis. Despite the fact that more research needs to be done, given what is now known, the future looks very bright for treating patients with PCOS.

Insulin resistance (which is a stepping stone on the path to diabetes) appears to be the key underlying abnormality in patients with PCOS. The many symptoms of PCOS provide us with an early warning system to the presence of insulin problems, even before we are able to detect laboratory abnormalities. Insulin resistance (particularly when unmasked at an early stage) is very treatable and provides the perfect opportunity to prevent diabetes and all of its complications, including hypertension and heart disease. Although more research is needed, existing data suggests there is great cause for optimism in women with PCOS.

A PERSONAL STORY

Pam

A PCOS diagnosis came for Pam when she was trying to conceive at around age thirty. "I always sort of knew something was wrong," she said. Her periods were regular as a teen, but then they started to get further and further apart. She went on birth-control pills for a while and her periods were regular during that time, but they were never right when she stopped taking the pill.

When she did try to get pregnant, Pam decided she was not going to stress about it. She was off the pill for several years, and for two years attempted to get pregnant with the idea that if it happened, it happened. She then went to an OB/GYN who did an ultrasound, and there on her ovaries were the classic cysts.

"I had had some of the other symptoms," Pam said, "hair growth and that kind of stuff but not severe; it was no big deal."

Her doctor recommended Clomid. It didn't work, and the doctor upped the dose three times, but Pam had trouble with side effects. "It made me feel like I was in a rage, so angry." For a long time Pam thought it was "just her," and resigned herself to the fact that she simply had a nasty personality. Then she talked with other women who had taken Clomid and had the same reaction, and she felt much better.

Pam then went to ovulation monitoring and used Metrodin to help her ovulate. After one cycle, tests showed that her estrogen level was too high, so her doctor prescribed Lupron to suppress the hormonal spikes, and after two cycles she got pregnant—and had twins.

The second time Pam wanted to conceive, they started right out with the Lupron, and she got pregnant with the first cycle. And Pam had triplets.

The twins are just starting school. Pam is no longer worried about conceiving again. She has more PCOS symptoms now since her children were born. Always on the heavier side, at 5'11" Pam now weighs more than her average 175 pounds, and she is often hypoglycemic.

Pam sought the help of an endocrinologist who was doing a study involving Glucophage and weight loss. "I didn't qualify for the study," Pam said, "but she saw me as a patient, and I pursued the study on my own with her." The endocrinologist prescribed Glucophage, and Pam dropped thirty pounds. "I felt so much better, no mood swings, no bouts of hunger."

She sees her endocrinologist approximately every six months. Pam is focusing on weight at the moment and would like to lose a few more pounds. She knows a better diet helps, and she tries to stay away from carbohydrates, "but it's hard."

Pam's family history includes diabetes and lots of heart disease. She attributes a lot of her success in controlling symptoms to the Glucophage regimen. Pam found she had to do a lot on her own to get to where she is, and she thinks that being a nurse helped her push through some medical barriers that may block other women with PCOS from getting the help they need in handling their symptoms.

And Pam laughs when she points out the fact that it took conceiving her twins and triplets to get her to this point with her own health.

CHAPTER ELEVEN ∾

Getting the Support You Need

PCOS is as individual as every woman who has this complex syndrome. That it is neither contagious nor, in and of itself, life-threatening does not lessen the fact that it is frustrating and complicated to manage.

Many of the side effects, as we have seen in previous chapters, have a significant impact on intimate relationships. Many of the symptoms are visible ones that can be embarrassing and add yet another level of stress that the PCOS patient has to confront. Adolescents with PCOS have to deal with these symptoms at a time when being teased and stigmatized is a crushing blow to self-esteem.

Symptoms are often so wide-ranging and seemingly unrelated that, even after diagnosis, women with polycystic ovarian syndrome are often misjudged. Many people have no idea what women who have PCOS are dealing with, and look upon them as hypochondriacs who are running to the doctor for minor inconveniences.

Combine all that with the simple fact that PCOS is not itself a disease and not even something that most people have ever heard of, and the roller-coaster ride that PCOS puts women on is quickly understandable.

Managing PCOS is difficult to go alone. As with any difficult issue in our lives, support from family, friends, and professionals is critical for success in managing PCOS. But first there is that huge hurdle to overcome: being believed when you claim that something is not quite right with your body.

You Are Not a Hypochondriac

Only you can decide how much detail you will share with family members and friends about your symptoms and PCOS diagnosis. You may have already become quite adept at hiding your more unusual visible symptoms, such as facial hair or thinning hair on your head, more typical of men than women. No one is likely to ask about acne, except perhaps your mother or your closest friend. More people than not are overweight in America, so you are perhaps happy to let friends, acquaintances, even family members think you are simply eating too much or not getting enough exercise—that's true for almost everyone, so why would anyone question it?

It's not that PCOS itself is a disorder that holds the social stigmas that have been attached to AIDS or sexually transmitted diseases. What does tend to happen, however, is that with such a multitude of seemingly unrelated symptoms, the woman with PCOS may in fact sound to some like a hypochondriac—there is always something wrong with her—if it isn't one thing one day, it's something else the next.

Women have long been accused of being melodramatic about the natural bodily changes that take place each month as the menstrual cycle ebbs and flows. Not until very recent times, perhaps within just a few decades, has it been understood and acknowledged that women do experience some dramatic physical issues with their menstrual cycles. While men have a tradition of avoiding their health and being concerned only when something significant happens—like a heart attack—and they can no longer avoid it, women tend toward being more proactive in their health care. However, they also have often been led to feel that they should be more stoic, that they are too emotional or make too much of things.

Nowadays, much more is known about the menstrual cycle and what can go wrong in the body's systems. As always, we live in the best of times and the worst of times. About some things, medical science knows just enough to make things more frustrating, but not enough to do anything concrete to remedy the situation. We are coming to understand many more diseases and conditions—fibromyalgia, PCOS, and Alzheimer's, to name just a few—but we still do not fully understand the root causes and therefore cannot proactively approach these conditions with confidence.

If you have been diagnosed with PCOS, now is the time to focus on managing it. Your health and well-being are in your hands. Easier said than done, for sure, but you cannot let other people, whoever they are and however well-intentioned they may be, lessen your concern with what is happening in your own body. Do not accept criticism for how you feel—your feelings are your feelings, and you have a right to them.

The best way to gain control of your feelings about this frustrating condition is to be proactive about diagnosis, care, treatment, and maintenance. Learn everything you can about this significant syndrome that is affecting your body.

Research—A First Step to the Support You Need

Stories abound of women who were repeatedly ignored by their family members and even doctors when they complained about a range of seemingly unrelated symptoms that they were experiencing. Many women tell of taking matters into their own hands and doing research that led them to the discovery of this condition called polycystic ovarian syndrome. When they stumbled across it in their research and read the symptoms, many women experienced the unbelievable feeling of having their own story right in front of their eyes. This tale of discovery is repeated over and over.

Many of these women also tell of still being patronized once they had this discovery in hand. Up until most recently, even many OB/GYNs either had not heard of PCOS or knew little about it. So even if their doctor agreed that they might have the syndrome, many women were still not getting concrete treatment.

If you are reading this book, you probably have already either been diagnosed or have discovered PCOS in your own research and suspect you have it. Don't stop there.

Continue to research any topics you find in this book that interest you. If a drug or treatment seems possibly helpful for you, based on your personal history, explore it. Discuss it with your doctor. If your doctor is not as helpful as you would like, find a new doctor who is willing to work with you. Second opinions are your right; as long as you deal with seeking a second opinion in a professional manner, your doctor should deal with it professionally as well. Second opinions are a common practice, and you should not be concerned about hurting your doctor's feelings. In fact, if you are seeing an OB/GYN, emphatically request a referral to an endocrinologist if you suspect or know you have PCOS.

The main way to get other people to provide you with the support you need and take this mysterious syndrome seriously is to take it seriously yourself and insist on the level of care that you need and deserve.

The Diabetes Connection

Many women have found that a frustrating element of a PCOS diagnosis is that people look at you blankly when you tell them what has finally been found out about your fertility issues or your seemingly disconnected collection of symptoms. Most people don't know about PCOS.

However, most people know about diabetes. This is where you can make the connection. We have learned that PCOS is a disorder of the endocrine system, as is diabetes. Your endocrine system regulates the hormones in your body and hormones are critical to the ability of your body to function well. Both PCOS and diabetes revolve around the hormone insulin.

Use the diabetes connection when you explain PCOS. While PCOS is not diabetes, recent research and discoveries seem to connect them as close cousins. We now know that many of the symptoms of PCOS are a direct result of insulin resistance, hyperinsulinemia, or hypoinsulinemia. The main keys to regulating both diabetes and PCOS are diet and exercise. Sometimes drug intervention is necessary, sometimes not. Maintaining appropriate glucose levels in the bloodstream is the watchword of all diabetics. And it becomes a critical component of PCOS management as well.

Lastly, there is a real connection with the fact that women with PCOS have a much higher likelihood of becoming diabetic. And gestational diabetes is often a factor in women with PCOS who become pregnant.

So when you go to explain PCOS to the doubtful or uninitiated, go ahead and use the diabetes comparison. You will probably find that instead of looking at you oddly, they will nod their heads in understanding. Sixteen million Americans have diabetes, meaning that almost everyone knows one or two people with diabetes and therefore has some passing knowledge of the disease. Use it to your advantage.

Depression

Women with PCOS can be high on the list for experiencing depression at some time during their attempts to manage their condition. It can be just from the seemingly overwhelming task of trying to control the various symptoms—that alone can sap your time and energy. Depression can be more severe for women who have experienced a long period of unsuccessful attempts to get pregnant. And for women who have symptoms that make relationships difficult, the lack of a partner and the accompanying feelings can be triggers for depression as well.

First, accept that depression is a very real thing, characterized by:

• Feeling down for more than a couple of days in a row
• Avoiding having a social life and preferring to stay at home by yourself
• Crying episodes without obvious provocation
• Persistent trouble sleeping
• Being overly critical of yourself
• Thinking about suicide, that the world/your family would be better off without you

If you have these classic signs, don't hesitate—pick up the phone and make an appointment with your doctor. Be frank with her or him about your feelings, and get a referral to a therapist or counselor who can help you work through these emotional downs.

Your doctor will also want to work with you on other possible causes of your depression. It may not be PCOS itself that is the culprit, but perhaps the medication you are on to treat one of the symptoms. The symptoms and treatments for PCOS can be overwhelming, and there are people who can help.

Sometimes, once you are diagnosed and get started on a plan to counteract PCOS, your new diet, with extra emphasis on good nutrition appropriate to your condition, or your exercise program can alone help perk your spirits. And these two things can also have such a huge impact on alleviating symptoms that the relief from annoying and embarrassing symptoms can also steer you off the road to depression.

Be kind to yourself. Now that you have a diagnosis and are taking care of your physical health, don't forget to take care of your mental and emotional health as well.

Pick-me-ups

Most women, thankfully, will not experience clinical depression as the result of PCOS. However, the complexity of this syndrome and your attempts to manage it will certainly, at some time or another, leave you feeling overwhelmed. There is a lot to learn and focus on— proper diet, often a whole new way of eating, and incorporating an exercise program. Whew, this is a lot for anyone! Top all that with a job, relationship, and family, and anyone would feel that she had quite a bit on her plate.

Don't forget to include little pick-me-ups and rewards in your day or week. If you really enjoy wine but have cut it out of your diet to control calorie count and sugar intake, treat yourself once in a while. Designate the first day of every month as the day you go out for a healthy salad and one glass of extremely good wine. Buy yourself a hardcover novel hot-off-the-press every time you meet a significant weight-loss goal—with the price of hardback fiction these days, this is a significant treat!

If you are working to incorporate exercise into your fairly sedentary life, treat yourself to a whole new hobby that will get you some of the exercise you need. For example:

> Take up birdwatching and come to look forward to weekend walks in the woods.

> Start taking horseback riding lessons at a local stable. Many adult women have found horseback riding to be a great workout and have turned to riding as a physical outlet. Many stables have created riding classes devoted to this demographic. Research the local stables carefully, and pick one that has a reputation for having kind, quiet school horses and a focus on safety.

> Buy a pair of inline skates and some protective gear, and join the young kids in the park; in winter, you can switch to iceskating.

> Rent a canoe on the weekends and explore a different waterway within short driving range from your home.

> Take up golf, tennis, bowling, beachcombing.

> If you don't tend to get outside or get exercise without some real motivation, consider something drastic, like getting a dog. Choose a breed appropriate to your lifestyle and home environment—yes, some dogs need a great amount of exercise and some less, but no matter what size the dog is, all dogs love walks! If you really get into

it, you can take the dog to obedience classes, and before you know it, you are involved in the great fun activity—for both you and your dog—of agility classes (in which dogs show their agility and obedience by going through tunnels, over fences, across bridges). You'll meet a whole new set of friends and have a hobby that is endless in its ability to give you something to look forward to.

Go to the library or bookstore and explore the outdoor recreation shelves for other ideas. There are lots of things you can do without spending much money. Some activities, like skating, require a one-time expenditure except for the occasional adjustment or roller replacement; every time you use the equipment after the initial purchase, it costs nothing additional. Some things, such as canoes, kayaks, and bicycles, can be rented, which holds the costs down and allows you to try sports out without having to own or store the equipment.

Relationship Issues

Some women interviewed for this book had put the idea of having an intimate relationship on hold while they tried to figure out what was going on with their bodies. Other women, who were already in a committed relationship and weren't experiencing much of the outward symptoms, discovered their PCOS diagnosis in the midst of attempting to get pregnant. Whatever the case with you, PCOS can take a toll on intimate relationships.

One woman interviewed said she got tired of her male partners thinking of her as "sick." After three partners, she finally gave up and put her intimate life on a way back burner.

If you have outward signs of PCOS such as excess facial hair and severe acne, it can be difficult feeling that you are going to be attractive to partners. When that is the case, it can help to plan to spend more time getting ready to go out for the evening. But remember, the most supportive partner is going to be the one who is attracted to your mind as well as your body—if a potential partner isn't supportive of something like your managing PCOS, you may find that person will not provide the support you need during other critical life-issues either.

Sex and PCOS

If your sex life is currently revolving around having a baby, this can be stressful indeed! For a woman with PCOS, it's a good idea to begin planning a family as early as possible. While few women in general know whether or not they are going to have fertility issues when they attempt to get pregnant, women with PCOS can expect it to be more difficult than it would be if they didn't have PCOS.

It can't be emphasized enough: Start managing your symptoms long before you think you may want to get pregnant. Then you are so much ahead of the game that you can avoid some of the intense time pressure.

Sex can also wane if you aren't feeling your best—emotionally or physically. Physical symptoms of PCOS can take their toll on a woman's desire to be intimate. Again, it may help to plan romance a little more. Perhaps by midweek, you and your partner can agree that on Saturday you will spend a romantic evening together. By planning, you can set aside some time on Saturday to concentrate on feeling your best. You can go to the extreme of going to the hairdresser for a great new do, or try something as simple as getting in a nice nap on Saturday afternoon so you won't feel so fatigued that evening. You want to look forward to some romance and sex, not feel as if it is a lot of work!

If you are finding sexual issues to be a real problem, don't ignore this. Sex is an important part of any committed relationship. Use books or therapists or videos or whatever works best for you to help your sexual relationship.

Don't just ignore it—any good relationship is worth it.

Support from Family

Your family will probably be your first line of support. If you have come to a PCOS diagnosis through the infertility channel, you will rely on your partner for a huge source of backup. He will know very well what you have gone through in trying to deal with PCOS-related symptoms. Combine the general symptoms with the stress of the pregnancy issue, and you will need a very supportive partner indeed.

The best way to be sure that you aren't getting overwhelmed all alone is to be upfront about things. Make a plan for starting a family, and don't put so much pressure on yourself that you can't possibly meet the goals you set up.

Sometimes it is helpful if your partner accompanies you to see your doctor to discuss PCOS, whether you are attempting to have children or not. It is simply a fact of life that a professional like a doctor can put a perspective on the situation that may make your partner—mother, sister, or any other family member you would find helpful—better understand what you are experiencing and alleviate any feelings they may have that you have become a hypochondriac.

Having a team member you can rely on during the worst of times is a key to dealing with the emotional side of this complex syndrome. Mom may know just the thing that is your favorite pick-me-up; your partner can know just how to help you stick to your diet or exercise regimen. Support from your loved ones is simply the best.

Support from Professionals

Expect all members of your health care team to take you seriously and be supportive of your decisions. If you do your research, keep up to date with the latest in PCOS (see Chapter Twelve for some ideas), and try to follow through with the management suggestions that your team members prescribe, they will respect you as the key player in your own medical team. Your family doctor, OB/GYN, dietitian, endocrinologist, personal trainer, and other practitioners should all be on your side, working together with you for the best results of your management plan.

Support from Friends

With any luck, you will have some close friends that you can share some of your PCOS experiences with. A true friend does not have to share your medical issues in order to be a shoulder to lean on. If you really want someone to help motivate you to get to the gym, ask your friends to be your exercise buddies. Tell them why it is important to your health and well-being, educate them about PCOS, and good friends will be there for you.

Support Groups

Many support groups are developing specifically for PCOS. You can find a couple of great ones online—PCOSA at pcosupport.org and SoulCysters at soulcysters.com are two that have very active chat groups and lots of research and information right on their sites.

PCOSA has local groups as well—check with them to find out if one exists in your area.

Check also with your local hospital. Many hospitals small and large provide informative support groups as part of their community outreach programs. Doctors are so busy and nurses are in such short supply that the role of support groups in patient education has become much more prominent.

Whether or not you have a partner, whether or not your family is close by, whether or not you can rely on any of them, or on your friends, to support you in your management of PCOS, support groups are out there. Talking with women who deal with the same issues you do can be both a relief and a motivation to keep up with the hard work involved in managing PCOS.

Getting the Word Out

The important thing is to get beyond feeling that you need to explain yourself to anyone else, and spend your time managing your condition instead. If anyone suggests that you are acting like a hypochondriac and that you don't need to see a doctor, learn how to smile and nod your head, then make an appointment.

Once you have a diagnosis, you can then choose how much to explain to your friends and family. Remember, the more people who know about PCOS, the less explaining you'll need to do. And the less explaining other women will need to do as well.

A PERSONAL STORY

Ashley

Ashley came to a PCOS diagnosis through the pregnancy route, like many of the other women who have told their personal stories in this book. When she and her husband decided they were ready to conceive, Ashley went off the pill. She started to gain weight and noticed a lot of skin-related changes and hair growth. She just kept gaining weight, and she had no cycles.

Her doctor told her it was probably just her body adjusting to her stopping the pill. He told her to wait six months.

One year later, Ashley had gained eighty pounds. She went back to her doctor, who told her she wasn't eating right or following her diet properly and put her on a diet plan. Ashley went to a new doctor.

She told her new doctor all her symptoms and said, "Something is going on." Within a few minutes, he suggested she had PCOS and sent her for an ultrasound and blood work. Sure enough, the classic cysts showed up on her ovaries. She also had a "dermoid cyst" on her ovary that needed to be removed. Ashley had surgery and for a few months cycled on her own then went back to no cycles.

She told her doctor that she really would like to get pregnant. The doctor suggested she concentrate on that and said that they would treat her PCOS after she had a baby. Ashley's next stop was a reproductive endocrinologist.

First she went on Provera, then Clomid for six months and got pregnant. "It was unbelievable," she says. Her daughter is now almost two years old.

After her daughter's birth, Ashley didn't do much for her PCOS for a few months, then her doctor started her on Glucophage. Her blood-sugar level came down, her cholesterol level came down, she lost twenty-four pounds, and she started to ovulate on her own. She had wanted to start trying to conceive again, but decided she wanted to concentrate on her own health. If she got pregnant, fine, and if not, that would be fine too.

"My daughter is a blessing," she says, "and I want to be around as long as possible." So her own health was a priority for her.

For Ashley, major lifestyle changes including diet and exercise have been a huge help in controlling the symptoms of PCOS. She has removed as much carbohydrates from her diet as possible without health implications. She is using the well-known "Zone" diet plan, eating lots of vegetables and proteins and excluding sugar from her diet as much as is possible.

Ashley also follows "The Firm" exercise program. This part-aerobic, part-weight-training program takes around one hour, and she can do it in her own home. Her attitude about fitting exercise into her day?

"If I can find close to twenty-three hours a day to do something for other people, I can find at least one hour to do something for myself."

CHAPTER TWELVE ∽

The Future

The topic of PCOS in the medical community is exploding with interest and research. Now that PCOS is more readily recognized and diagnosed, and the links between PCOS and insulin have begun to be documented and studied, you can expect an exponential increase in the rate of study of PCOS and the knowledge that is gained. This can only be good news for the woman with PCOS.

Clinical Trials

One way you can get involved in the future of PCOS is to become involved in clinical trials. This is not something for everyone, but for those with a "help others" attitude and a strong interest in research of their own conditions, clinical trials can be very interesting at the least and very helpful to your own experience with symptoms at best.

There are many ways to find out about upcoming clinical trials. Several Web sites keep updated lists and give detailed information about the trial and the kinds of participants they are seeking. Check:

- *National Institutes of Health:* The government-funded health research institutes provide a Web site (www.clinicaltrials.gov) that identifies health-related research studies. One interesting thing about this site is that you can find information even about clinical trials that are no longer recruiting for participants.

- *CenterWatch:* You can search the CenterWatch site (www.center-watch.com) by condition. A search of PCOS called up fifteen clinical trials taking place all over the country, from Arizona to Massachusetts, Florida, New Mexico, Montana, and many states in between. CenterWatch also has a patient-notification service that will keep you posted on up to twenty conditions that you have selected. And all information remains confidential.

You can also find PCOS-specific clinical trials listed on PCOS Web sites such as PCOSA (pcosupport.org) and SoulCysters (SoulCysters.com).

Studies

A study conducted by at the University of Alabama was listed as "Prevalence of polycystic ovarian syndrome in unselected black and white women in the southeastern United States: A Prospective Study."

The study showed that 25 percent of women showing polycystic ovaries are asymptomatic. "A more comprehensive definition of PCOS arose from a conference on the disorder in April 1990, sponsored by the NIH/NICHHD. Although a clear-cut consensus was never reached, the majority of participants believed that PCOS should be defined by 1) ovulatory dysfunction 2) clinical evidence of hyperandrogenism (hirsutism, acne, androgenic alopecia) and/or hyperandrogenemia, and 3) exclusion of related disorders."

The conclusion of the study was "...the overall prevalence of PCOS appears to be approximately 4.6%, although it could be as low as 3.5% and as high as 11.2%, using the NIH/NICHHD 1990 criteria. There appeared to be no significant difference in prevalence between white and black women. Our data support the concept that PCOS is one of the most common reproductive endocrinological disorders of women."

Armed with this kind of information, you can feel more in control of your condition, just by knowing that there is a high prevalence and that there are studies being done. You can also become aware of treatments that may help you and your specific symptoms. You can consult with your doctor more thoroughly, being more informed. And last but not least, you can feel self-assured as you talk with skeptical friends and family members who have not heard of and do not understand PCOS.

Some of the other topics currently under study through clinical trials are:

• Interaction of androgens and opioids in PCOS
• Effects of luteinizing hormone on androgen secretion in PCOS
• PCOS and sleep-disordered breathing
• The combination of a new insulin sensitizing medication, rosiglitazone, taken along with clomiphrene to induce ovulation

Information on these studies can be found at the various clinical trial Web sites.

Participating in a clinical trial may or may not be right for you. Maybe you have some parameters that you would be okay with—you'd participate in a trial that involves a drug as long as the drug has already been approved by the FDA, for instance.

Some clinical trials may take you away from home for several days to a couple of weeks or more, although this is not often a requirement of the trial—it is more a factor of where the trial is taking place in relation to your home. If you live near a large urban area where there are many large medical facilities, or if you live near a university where research is always taking place, you may find something nearby, but if you live in a rural setting it narrows the possibilities quite a bit.

Clinical trials are carefully regulated—any study needs to be reviewed and approved by the Institutional Review Board, which includes both physicians and laypeople, who bring the participant's perspective to the review process.

The CenterWatch and NIH sites both outline the specifics of how to get involved in a clinical trial. Some questions they recommend asking about any study include:

> Who is the sponsor of the trial? Often this will be a large pharmaceutical company or the NIH or some other government organization. Don't be overly suspicious if the trial is being sponsored by a drug company—they are under extremely tight regulations and scrutiny by federal government agencies.

> Are there any costs to me for the trial? If you have to travel to the trial site and stay in a hotel for the duration, who is responsible for the costs? If you have to travel quite a distance everyday for the trial, who pays for that commuting cost? If you live next door

to the Mayo Clinic, you have a leg up on the chance that an appropriate clinical trial on PCOS will be in your neighborhood—
but that convenience is rare.

Exactly what treatment(s) are going to be used? Drugs, alternative treatments? Will there be x-rays involved? How will the drugs
be administered?

Some of the answers to your questions will easily be found in the literature provided about the study, especially from a form called an "informed consent form." As the title of the form implies, it reviews the
study, what the patient can expect to have happen to her during the
study, and any risks that may be involved in participating in this study—
drug side effects, and so forth. Also, keep in mind that it is within your
rights to opt out of the clinical trial at any time during the process.

You should also plan to discuss your participation with your medical
team. Have your doctor review the information about the study and go
over it with you. If she or he has any questions or concerns, they should
be answered. Clinical trials usually have a contact person, such as a
research assistant, to handle your questions.

Once you understand the details of the study, you need to sign the
informed consent form, which states that you have now been fully
informed and are signing your approval to participate.

Drug Testing

Pharmaceutical companies are always researching drugs to fight the
old and new diseases and conditions that human beings suffer. Sometimes they are not inventing new drugs but are simply looking for new
uses for existing drugs. However, drugs are approved only for a specific

use—if there are other possible uses for the drug, they need to go through the entire approval process.

The good thing about new uses for existing drugs is that a lot is already known about the side effects of the drug on human beings. New drugs will have had years of testing on laboratory animals, but what a drug does to a mouse is not necessarily what it will do to a human being.

In order to test new drugs on human beings, the pharmaceutical company has to go through a complex four-phase process. According to CenterWatch, the process goes like this:

> *Phase One:* This initial phase is focused on safety. What does the drug do to a healthy human being? What happens as the dose is increased? The people in the study are carefully monitored to find out exactly how the body processes the drug at the different dosage levels. These studies often pay the participants.

> *Phase Two:* This phase concentrates on the effectiveness of the drug. This phase can last up to a couple of years, typically has several hundred participants, and is what is known as "blind"— part of the group gets the drug, part of the group gets a placebo, and no one, researcher or patient, knows who is getting what. About 70 percent of drugs tested in Phase One get to Phase Two.

> *Phase Three:* Phase Three drug study is intense, lasting over several years and involving at least several hundred and perhaps several thousand participants. Around a third of the drugs pass through Phase Two and make it to this critical stage. The drug is thoroughly put through its paces for all aspects of success, side effects, and effectiveness in treating the condition it is being tested for. This phase costs the pharmaceutical company

developing the drug lots of money and lots of time, so it is not surprising that up to 90 percent of drugs making it to this phase pass on to the final phase of study.

Phase Four: This phase takes on a different look and begins to compare the drug with other therapies already being prescribed for the condition, including other drugs as well as other types of nondrug treatments (physical therapy, surgery, etc.). Having gone through the first three phases, the drug can also be monitored for long-term effects, both beneficial and negative.

Clinical trials are interesting. With a condition such as PCOS, it can be very exciting to see what is coming down the pike for possible treatments. Because much of PCOS treatment involves treating the symptoms, you may find that a lot of the trials will involve testing other purposes for an existing drug, or that they don't involve drugs at all, since many of the PCOS symptoms already have clearly defined drug therapies.

The idea of participating in a clinical trial may not be for you. One woman we interviewed for this book was about to leave for six days to participate in a clinical trial that was focused on the effects of diet and exercise on women with PCOS. She was understandably reluctant to leave her children for that long, for the first time ever, but she also was excited about participating. Participation included an intense follow-up of several months, during which she would get complete handholding for her diet and exercise regimen. She was also excited that the results of the trial might help other women with PCOS.

When you monitor what is on the horizon for treatment that has entered the clinical trial process, you are armed with more knowledge about what to discuss with your doctor, in attempting to treat your symptoms.

Clearly, the future of PCOS involves further study of the relationship of insulin to the syndrome. This now-accepted aspect of PCOS is a relatively new link, so what is over the horizon can only be imagined!

Because of the insulin connection, women with PCOS would do well to also follow the research in diabetes care and treatment. The good news/bad news here is that these two conditions affect so many people (over 16 million Americans with diabetes and an average of 5 percent of American women with PCOS) that they will not be ignored in the medical community.

Your Future and PCOS

If you have read this far in this book, you are among the women committed to making their lives better. For some women, the effects of PCOS are simply annoying and sometimes embarrassing, and for the most part to be ignored. But the case for not ignoring PCOS is manifold:

> First and foremost, the long-term consequences of PCOS on a woman's body are largely unknown. It is critical for your good health not to risk ignoring the symptoms of PCOS and the implications they may have for your future health and well-being, and the quality of life of both you and your family. PCOS can offer you an opportunity to take the steps necessary to prevent diabetes. Believe it or not, this is a gift, an opportunity that should not be wasted.

> The treatments for the individual symptoms of PCOS abound. You do not have to "suffer through" the symptoms that affect your self-esteem. From most of the women with PCOS that we talked with, we heard the lament that lack of periods, male-pattern hair growth, and acne make them "feel not quite a

woman." Don't ignore such feelings, because these conditions are treatable—some more easily than others, but nonetheless there are things you can do.

You can be a role model for your kids: teach them by example to take good care of themselves and their overall health. It's good for them and appreciated by those who love them.

We wish you all the best in your pursuit of good health!

A PERSONAL STORY

Cindy

From the time she started her period, Cindy was never regular; and by late high school her cycles were gone completely. She never told anyone until she entered college and went to the campus doctor for something unrelated. The doctor noticed she had an unusual amount of hair growth and mentioned that her symptoms were not quite right.

She went to an endocrinologist to start searching for an answer. And search they did—with urine tests, adrenal gland tests, and tests she can't even recall. Cindy was checked for conditions such as Cushing's syndrome and other genetic issues.

Finally she got a diagnosis of Stein-Leventhal syndrome, aka PCOS, and compared to all of the ominous things that she was being tested for, this seemed relatively minor. She was put on birth-control pills, and this seemed to take care of a lot.

Three years after Cindy got married, she and her husband wanted to have a baby, and Cindy found herself at a fertility clinic. She started with Clomid, went to injections, and got pregnant. Sadly, she miscarried at five months.

After bumping around to various insurance companies, she was on her last chance. She talked with her doctor about the protocol her friend with PCOS was on, and although the doctor indicated that it was not a protocol they used, Cindy was insistent. And soon pregnant. And she now has a five-year-old son.

Hair growth has perhaps been one of the most troublesome issues for Cindy, right from adolescence. She has done electrolysis for years and years, and in the beginning was doing as much as four hours per week. The electrolysis has worked, and now she goes perhaps twice a year. "It's expensive and it takes time, but it does work. I was more bothered by it in my early twenties, when appearance is everything."

Cindy happened to find out about the PCOS/insulin connection while doing research on the Internet. She mentioned it to her doctor, who said she would check it out. The doctor happened to be attending a diabetes convention shortly after this discussion, and came back excited to have learned more about the insulin/PCOS connection that Cindy had alerted her to. Cindy went on Glucophage to control her insulin and blood sugar, and things have changed. She feels much better and much more in control of her PCOS.

Cindy is one of the small percentage of women with PCOS for whom weight is not a major issue. However, lately she wanted to lose some weight and began following a diet that lowered her carbohydrate intake. She lost twenty pounds and feels much better.

PCOS is not much of a factor in Cindy's life these days. "When I was trying to have a child," she said, "PCOS consumed me. At this point in my life, it doesn't impact me all that much."

GLOSSARY

Acanthosis nigricans: Dark and velvety skin, usually on the back of the neck and under the breasts, thought to be associated with insulin resistance.

Acrochordons: Skin tags.

Actos: An insulin-sensitizing drug that allows the insulin in your body to work more effectively (generic name: pioglitazone).

Adrenal gland: Gland that releases DHEA (dehydroepiandrostenedione) hormone and other androgens, as well as the stress hormones cortisol and adrenalin.

Aldactone: A testosterone receptor blocking medication for use in inhibiting testosterone receptors in cells from being stimulated by testosterone (generic name: spironolactone).

Alopecia: Hair loss.

Amen: A synthetic progesterone used to treat progesterone deficiency, in order to thicken the lining of the uterus and promote shedding of the endometrium (generic name: medroxyprogesterone).

Amenorrhea: Absence of menstrual periods.

Amino acids: Building blocks found in proteins that help build, repair, and maintain tissue.

Androgens: Male hormones (such as androstendione, DRIEA, and testoserone).

Anorexia nervosa: A serious eating disorder whereby the person starves herself, potentially to death.

Anovulation: Lack of ovulation.

Avandia: An insulin-sensitizing drug that allows the insulin in your body to work more effectively (generic name: rosiglitazone).

Bariatric surgery: Controlling weight by surgery.

Bioidentical: Synthetic compounds chemically indistinguishable from compounds produced by the human body.

Bulimia: A serious eating disorder characterized by binging then purging through vomiting.

Cilia: Hairlike fibers on the fallopian tube lining that help move the egg along.

Clomid: An ovulation-inducing drug (generic name: clomiphene).

Contraindicated: Term for a drug or treatment that is not recommended for a certain category of patient.

Corpus luteum: The empty follicle that once held the egg before ovulation.

Cycrin: A synthetic progesterone used to treat progesterone deficiency, in order to thicken the lining of the uterus and promote shedding of the endometrium (generic name: medroxyprogesterone).

Cysts: Masses in ovaries, breasts, and elsewhere that are often filled with fluid and are often benign.

Diabetes: A condition in which the body either does not use insulin efficiently or does not produce insulin at all, resulting in abnormal blood-sugar levels.

Dutasteride: A soon-to-be-released new testosterone metabolism blocker.

Dysmenorrhea: Painful periods.

Endocrinologist: A specialist of the endocrine system, the body system that controls all hormonal secretion and function.

Endometrium: The lining of the uterus.

Enzymes: Complex proteins found in the bloodstream and tissue.

Eulexin: One of the strongest antiandrogen medications available; can have serious side effects (generic name: flutamide).

Fallopian tubes: The part of the woman's reproductive anatomy where the egg travels to meet the sperm, be fertilized, and get to the uterus.

Fimbriae: The fringed ends of the fallopian tubes.

Follicle: The sac in the ovary that contains an egg (there are hundreds).

Follistim: An ovulation-inducing drug (generic name: FSH).

FSH: Follicle-stimulating hormone, the hormone that tells the ovary follicle to release an egg.

Glucophage: An insulin-sensitizing drug that allows the insulin in your body to work more effectively (generic name: metformin).

Glucose: Food is digested and converted to glucose, which is also called blood sugar and is a source of energy.

Glycemic index: The measure of how a standard number of calories from a given food impacts blood sugar. The faster a food is digested and the more calories it contains, the more the blood-sugar level will spike.

Glyset: An "insulin-sparing" agent that inhibits the enzyme needed to digest carbohydrates (generic name: miglitol).

Gonal F: An ovulation-inducing drug (generic name: FSH).

Hirsutism: Excess male-type hair growth in women.

Humegon: An ovulation-inducing drug (generic name: menotropins).

Hyperinsulinemia: Elevated insulin levels.

Hyperprolactinemia: Excess of the hormone prolactin, which stimulates production of breast milk.

Hypoglycemia: Low levels of blood sugar.

Hypothalamus: A major control center of the brain that regulates the endocrine and nervous systems.

Hyperthyroidism: Condition characterized by an overactive thyroid.

Hypothyroidism: Condition characterized by an underactive thyroid.

Insulin: A hormone secreted by the pancreas that controls blood-sugar levels.

IVF: In vitro fertilization; process by which an egg is fertilized in the laboratory and then inserted back into the womb.

LH: Luteinizing hormone, which is released by the pituitary gland and causes ovulation.

Laparoscopy: Surgical method involving the use of a tube with a camera on the end, known as a laparoscope.

Lupron: A drug often used as part of an infertility treatment program to prepare the ovaries for better response to ovulation-inducing medications (generic name: leuprolide).

Menorrhagia: Heavy-flowing period.

Menstruation: The onset of the shedding of the uterine lining.

Neonatologist: A doctor specializing in newborns.

Oligomenorrhea: Irregular periods.

Ovaries: The organs of the female reproductive system that store and release eggs.

Ovulation: The release of an egg from the ovary.

Pancreas: Gland that releases insulin.

Pergonal: An ovulation-inducing drug (generic name: menotropins).

Pituitary gland: Signals release of hormones, including estrogen.

Precose: An "insulin-sparing" agent that inhibits the enzyme needed to digest carbohydrates (generic name: acarbose).

Pregnyl: An ovulation-inducing drug (generic name: hCG).

Profasi: An ovulation-inducing drug (generic name: hCG).

Prometrium: A bioidentical progesterone used to treat progesterone deficiency, in order to thicken the lining of the uterus and promote shedding of the endometrium (generic name: progesterone).

Propecia: Drug known as a testosterone metabolism blocker that prevents conversion of less active testosterone to a strong, more active form (generic name: finasteride).

Prostaglandins: Chemicals that signal the uterine lining to begin shedding.

Provera: A synthetic progesterone used to treat progesterone deficiency, in order to thicken the lining of the uterus and promote shedding of the endometrium (generic name: medroxyprogesterone).

Repronex: An ovulation-inducing drug (generic name: menotropins).

Rogaine: An over-the-counter hair-growth stimulator (generic name: minoxidil).

Serophene: An ovulation-inducing drug (generic name: clomiphene).

SHBG: Sex-hormone-binding globulin.

Stein-Leventhal syndrome: The original name for PCOS, after the two doctors who first diagnosed it.

Tagamet: A testosterone receptor blocking medication for use in inhibiting testosterone receptors in cells from being stimulated by testosterone (generic name: cimetidine).

TSH: Thyroid-stimulating hormone.

Uterus: The organ of the female reproductive system where the fetus develops.

Vaniqa: A cream that slows unwanted facial hair growth (generic name: eflornithine).

BIBLIOGRAPHY

Balch, James F., M. D. and Phyllis Balch, C.N.C. *Prescription for Nutritional Healing,* second edition. Garden City, NY: Avery Publishing Group 1997.

Balen, Adam. "Pathogenesis of polycystic ovary syndrome—the enigma unravels?" *The Lancet.* September 18 1999 v354 n9183 p966.

Boston Women's Health Collective. *Our Bodies, Ourselves for the New Century.* New York: Touchstone 1998.

Bryan, Brenda. "Insulin Resistance." *PCOS Bulletin* Fall 2001.

Cheskin, Lawrence J., M.D. and Ron Sauder. *New Hope for People with Weight Problems.* New York: Prima 2002.

Cooper, Nancy. *The Convenience Foods Cookbook.* Minneapolis: IDC Publishing 1998.

Couzin, Jennifer. "It's not your fault: A deceptive disorder known as PCOS makes women feel guilty about obesity and some peculiar health problems." *Newsweek.* November 5 2001 p70.

Duyff, Roberta. *The American Dietetic Association's Complete Food and Nutrition Guide.* New York: Wiley 1998.

Eshref, H. *Easy Exercise to Relieve Stress.* Avon, MA: Adams Media 1999.

Francis-Cheung, Theresa. *A Break in Your Cycle: The Medical and Emotional Causes and Effects of Amenorrhea*. Minneapolis: Chronimed 1998.

Francis-Cheung, Theresa. *A Woman's Guide to Staying Healthy Through Her 30s*. Avon, MA: Adams Media 2002.

Franz, Marion J. *Fast Food Facts,* fifth edition. Minneapolis: IDC Publishing 1998.

Glenville, Marilyn, PhD. *The Nutritional Health Handbook for Women*. London: Piatkus 2001.

Goggins, Kim. "Looking for PCOS." *Chatelaine* May 2002 v75 n5 p74.

Greener, Mark. "Metaformin finds new role in PCOS pregnancies." *Pharmaceutical Business News*. March 20 2002 n410 p22.

"Happy Ending." *Woman's World*. May 28 2002 p13.

Harris, Colette with Dr. Adam Carey. *PCOS: A Woman's Guide to Dealing with Polycystic Ovarian Syndrome*. London: Thorsons 2000.

Harris, Colette with Theresa Cheung. *PCOS Diet Book*. London: Thorsons 2002.

Jancin, Bruce. "Campaign aims to redefine PCOS as endocrine disorder." *Family Practice News*. August 15 2000 v30 n16 p1.

Jancin, Bruce. "Effect of PCOS on cardiac risk remains controversial." *Family Practice News*. August 15 2000 v30 n16 p2.

Jancin, Bruce. "Hyperinsulinemia, not ovaries, at core of PCOS." *Family Practice News.* Jan 15 2001 v31 n2 p26.

Jancin, Bruce. "Metformin appears effective in teens with PCOS." *Family Practice News.* August 15 2000 v30 n16 p4.

Jancin, Bruce. "PCOS not linked to increased coronary risk." *Family Practice News.* June 15 2000 v30 n12 p30.

Jancin, Bruce. "Test all PCOS patients for thyroid disease." *Family Practice News.* October 1 2001 v31 n19 p1.

Kirn, Timothy F. "U.S. prevalence of PCOS is estimated at 6%." *Family Practice News* August 15 2002 v32 n16.

Levine, Hallie. "5 Down-There Diseases You Don't Know About But Should." *Glamour* May 2002 p127.

Lieberman, Shari and Nancy Bruning. *The Real Vitamin & Mineral Book,* second edition. Garden City Park, NY: Avery Publishing Group 1997.

Magee, Elaine. *The Good News Eating Plan for Type II Diabetes.* New York: Wiley 1998.

Magill's Medical Guide, Volume II. Revised Edition. Pasadena, CA: Salem Press, Inc. 1998.

Mindell, Earl. *Earl Mindell's Supplement Bible.* New York: Simon & Schuster 1998.

Monthly Nutrition Companion. Minneapolis: Chronimed 1997.

Murray, Michael and Joseph Pizzorno. *Encyclopedia of Natural Medicine,* second edition. Rocklin, CA: Prima Publishing 1998.

Northrup, Christiane, M.D. *Women's Bodies, Women's Wisdom.* New York: Bantam 1994.

Paolucci, Michelle. "Hide and Seek." *Nurseweek.com.*

Puffer, Paula. "A Hairy Issue: Dealing with Hirsutism." *OBGYN.net.*

Sattar, Naveed, Zoe E.C. Hopkinson, and Ian A Greer. "Insulin-sensitising agents in polycystic-ovary syndrome." *The Lancet.* January 13 1998 v351 n9099 p305.

Shimer, Porter. *New Hope for People with Diabetes.* New York: Prima 2001.

Snacking Habits for Healthy Living. Minneapolis: Chronimed 1997.

Thatcher, Samuel S., M.D., Ph.D. *PCOS: The Hidden Epidemic.* Indianapolis, IN: Perspectives Press 2000.

Thompson, Douglass S., M.D., ed. *Every Woman's® Health: The complete guide to body and mind.* New York: Doubleday 1993.

Trent, Maria E., Michael Rich, S. Bryn Austin, and Catherine M. Gordon. "Quality of life in adolescent girls with polycystic ovary syndrome." *Archives of Pediatrics & Adolescent Medicine.* June 2002 v156 n6 p55.

Ullman, Dana. *The Consumer's Guide to Homeopathy.* New York: Putnam 1995.

Webb, Marcus A. *The Herbal Companion*. Allentown, PA: People's Medical Society 1997.

"What Is Polycystic Ovarian Syndrome?" *MayoClinic.com*.

Wilde, Clare. *Hands-On Energy Therapy*. North Pomfret, VT: Trafalgar Square Publishing 1999.

Wills, Judith. *Four Weeks to Total Energy*. London: Quadrille 2000.

Woodham, Anne and Dr. David Peters. *Encyclopedia of Healing Therapies*. New York: Dorling Kindersley 1997.

Wright, Audrey, Sandra Nissenberg, and Betsy Manis. *Foods to Stay Vibrant, Young, and Healthy*. Minneapolis: Chronimed 1995.

Yeager, Selene. *The Doctor's Book of Food Remedies*. Emmaus, PA: Rodale Press 1998.

INDEX

T

Tagamet, 92

tai chi, 139, 167, 181-182

teenagers, 27-28, 59

testing, *see* diagnosis

testosterone, *see* androgens

thiazolidinediones, 94

thinness, menstruation and, 61.

    see also weight control

thyroid disorders, 187-188

thyroid-stimulating hormone (TSH),

    189-190

Tomer, Dr. Yaron, 21

traditional Chinese medicine (TCM),

    see energy therapies

Type 2 diabetes, *see* diabetes (type 2)

U

United States Department of Agriculture,

    dietary guidelines, 115-116

United States Pharmocopeia, 174

uterus, 34

V

Vaniqa cream, 96, 99

vitamins, 114, 161, 169, 173

W

walking, 135, 136

water, 114-115, 118

wedge resection, *see* surgery, for PCOS cysts

weight control

    benefits of, 98, 133

    body shape and, 107-109

    causes of weight gain, 108-107

    central obesity, 24

    drug therapies and, 54-55, 98-99,

        100-101, 121-122

    importance of, 107-108

infertility and, 66, 67, 154

menstruation and, 39, 61-62, 158-159

nutrition and, 55-57

PCOS symptoms and, 26, 144-145

problems with, 53-58

psychology of, 123-126

surgery for, 57, 123

unhealthy methods of, 58, 108

weight-loss franchises, 120-121

see also exercise; nutrition

weight-training, 141-142

Weight Watchers, 120-121

Wild, Dr. Sarah H., 16

X

Xenical, 98

Y

yin and yang, 179, 180, 181-182

yoga, 140, 167, 175-176

ACKNOWLEDGMENTS

Cheryl Kimball's energy and enthusiasm are what made this book possible. Thank you, Cheryl! The incredible support of Joanie and Matt, my wife and son, is what allows me to write. I owe them thanks and love—big time. The persistence and wisdom of my patients in seeking out elusive answers to their health challenges (sometimes with my help, and sometimes despite my help) are both inspiring and humbling. Thanks to all of you.

—M.H.

The people whom I have met, either in person, over the phone, or via e-mail, who are somehow personally involved in PCOS are some of the kindest, most caring people I've ever been privileged to associate with. I have a few specific ones to thank:

First, I would like to thank my coauthor, Dr. Milton Hammerly. He is a professional in the purest sense of the word—timely, responsive, committed, and all with good humor and grace.

A ton of thanks go to my friend, horseback riding pal, and "pinch" writer/editor/researcher, Sue Ducharme. Sue's good work is behind the thoroughness of the "Alternative Treatments" and "How Things Should Work" chapters in this book.

Many thanks go to Carol Arnold, Marketing Director of PCOSA, the online support group (www.pcosupport.org). Carol was on board from the moment I first e-mailed her. Her commitment is inspiring, and her assistance in many aspects of this book is much appreciated. Thanks also to the PCOSA Founder, Christine DeZarn, who graciously and enthusiastically agreed to write the foreword.

Thanks, also, to my sister-in-law, Susan Kline, who provided me with some interview prospects and helped move this book along. And thanks so much to all the women who allowed me to pry into their personal lives and interview them. Their stories are amazing, these women are amazing, and I wish them all the best in the world.

And last, but certainly not least, thanks to editor Paula Munier, who got me into this, and to Wendy Simard, the magician otherwise known as a "developmental editor," as well as everyone else at Fair Winds Press. They have been patient and kind during the creation of this manuscript. They recognized a topic that needed more voice in the world of women's health, explained in a way that was supportive and readable, not clinical and complicated. I commend Fair Winds for adding this book to their publishing program.

Acknowledgment sections are usually written at the end of the creation of a manuscript, and such is the case with this one. It's been a long haul and, to be honest, I wish I had at least six more months to continue to research and write about this complex condition. But all books must come to an end, so I think I'm going to just go take a nap.

—C.K.